FINDING HOPE IN THE LIVED EXPERIENCE OF PSYCHOSIS

This book offers first-person accounts of the experience of psychosis from the inside and the outside, through the eyes of two doctors, one of whom has experienced psychosis and both of whom have worked for decades in the field of psychiatry.

Underpinned by rigorous academic analysis using an evocative duo-ethnographic approach, the book explores the cultural and subcultural influences from childhood onwards – both traumatic and resilience-building – that have shaped their lives. Both authors reflect on strategies they learned early in life for dealing with challenges, each managing to function at a high level while avoiding awareness of their vulnerability. They reflect on the potential dangers of using their expertise and position of power in psychiatry simply to diagnose mental illness and prescribe medication. The differences and similarities in the authors' stories provide a productive tension highlighting the complexities of this paradigm shift that is happening in psychiatry.

Written in the form of two interacting memoirs, this book is of great interest to researchers, clinicians, and practicing psychologists, as well as a general audience with interest in psychosis.

Patte Randal, LRPC, MRCS, DPhil, has personal experience of recovery from psychosis. Her published research includes evaluation of a therapeutic intervention she developed for people with treatment refractory psychosis, and qualitative exploration of doctors' experience of mental health care. Retired from 30 years of clinical practice, she now promotes the implementation of 'The Gift Box', a collaborative resilience-building tool based on her 'Re-covery' model.

Josephine Stanton, MA, MBChB, FRANZCP, is a psychiatrist working with adolescents, children, mothers and babies and their families. Her research has included qualitative studies of mothers who have killed their children, experiences of doctors who have become patients of psychiatrists, and referrers and young people's experience of engaging with an acute inpatient unit.

THE INTERNATIONAL SOCIETY FOR PSYCHOLOGICAL AND SOCIAL APPROACHES TO PSYCHOSIS BOOK SERIES

Series editor: Anna Lavis

The International Society for Psychological and Social Approaches to Psychosis (ISPS) comprises a diverse range of individuals, networks and institutional members across more than twenty countries. Central to its ethos is that the perspectives of individuals with lived experience of psychosis, and their families and friends, are key to forging more inclusive understandings of, and collaborative therapeutic approaches to, psychosis.

With a core aim of promoting psychological and social approaches to psychosis, ISPS has a history stretching back more than five decades. During this time it has witnessed the relentless pursuit of primarily biological explanations for psychosis. This tide has been turning in recent years, with growing international recognition of a range of psychological, social, and cultural factors that have considerable explanatory traction and distinct therapeutic possibilities. Policymakers, treatment professionals, people with lived experience of psychosis, and family members are increasingly exploring interventions in which talking and listening are key ingredients. Psychosocially informed understandings and support frameworks are helpful for fostering and promoting personal recovery in the face of adverse psychotic experience. Recognising the humanitarian and therapeutic potential of these perspectives, ISPS embraces a wide spectrum of approaches from psychodynamic, systemic, cognitive, and arts therapies, to need-adapted and dialogical approaches, family and group therapies and residential therapeutic communities.

A further ambition of ISPS is to draw together diverse viewpoints on psychosis and to foster discussion and debate across the biomedical and social sciences, including establishing meaningful dialogue with practitioners and researchers who are more familiar with biological-based approaches. Such discussions are supported by growing evidence of the entanglement of genes and physiology with socio-cultural, environmental, and emotional contexts. This allows a consideration of mental distress as an embodied psycho-social experience that must be understood in relation to a person's life history and circumstances.

The ISPS book series seeks to capture these developments in the field by providing a forum in which authors with a variety of lived and professional

'A big takeaway from this book is the inequitable clash of world views when a person with lived experience of mental distress enters the sanctum of mainstream psychiatry. As a psychiatric registrar Patte Randal used her lived experience to foster connection, meaning and hope while many of her colleagues were steeped in psychiatric pessimism, biological reductionism, risk management and the use of force. Patte paid a heavy price but persisted for decades and triumphed with recovery affirming approaches that, unlike much of mainstream psychiatry, honour the etymology of her profession as "healers of the soul"'.

Mary O'Hagan, Former Mental Health Commissioner;
Author of Madness Made Me

'This book is remarkable for its scope, its honesty and directness. Dr. Randal's life covers so many different perspectives on psychosis and extreme experiences. She has built on Laing's recognition of finding meaning and the value of human contact for people with psychosis. Through her personal adventures and academic research she has inspired others, including her co-author and interviewer Dr. Stanton, and also built a teaching resource in this complex field. Dr. Stanton describes her own journey and helps link us to other positive developments in psychiatric therapy. If life is a "gigantic cosmic jig-saw puzzle" then this inspiring book may help you find solutions'.

Nick Argyle, MRCPsych, FRANZCP, Psychiatrist in Australasia working with
refugees: Formerly Clinical Director Auckland District Health Board

'This book contains the stories of two remarkable women doctors. Their courage and commitment to all they serve, and themselves, shines out of every page. I have been privileged to work alongside them both over many years and I have witnessed their dedication to challenging the traditional practice of psychiatry to be more humanistic and healing. I have learnt more from Patte than from any professional development I have ever attended. They have both walked the walk and have been punished for not submitting to the dominant discourse. Nevertheless, they have persisted and this book is a tribute to their determination and perseverance; as is 'The Gift Box', which I believe is a valuable resource for any service that is genuinely interested in promoting growth and self-development'.

Debbie Antcliff, FRANZCP, Retired Psychiatrist:
Formerly Clinical Director Buchanan Rehabilitation Centre;
Director of Area Mental Health Services Auckland District Health Board

'"*Finding Hope in the Lived Experience of Psychosis*" provides readers with a unique perspective on paths to recovery. The authors bring out the knowledge and insight that come both from personal experience with psychosis and from professional careers as doctors working in psychiatry. Their exploration of psychosis and extreme states makes for an evocative read'.

Robert Whitaker, Author of Anatomy of an Epidemic

'The beautiful story-telling stands out in this honest, rich and moving dual account of psychosis viewed from the inside and the outside. Written by two women doctors, trained in psychiatry, this unique evocative book provides a window into a deeply personal experience, and enriches the literature in this complex field'.

Patrick McGorry, Executive Director Orygen Youth Health Research Centre and Professor of Youth Mental Health at University of Melbourne

'In this lucidly written dual autobiography, two women, each of gifts and understanding, explore their personal experience of the conceptual fault line that runs through the theory and practice of psychiatry – the fault line dividing lived experience and objective clinical science, mind and soma, faith and scepticism, the numinous and the mundane, compassion and dispassion. They trace their stumbles along this line, their agonies, their triumphant successes and attendant dangers. I played a minor part in the saga of Patte – evidently not on the side of the angels – and recall the hard problems posed for her senior colleagues in doing her justice. I recommend this book to trainees and teachers in psychiatry. Let them read, and consider how they straddle the fault line'.

JJ Wright, Honorary Professor, Department of Psychological Medicine, University of Auckland School of Medicine

'This moving and thought-provoking book is built around the autobiographical accounts of two women doctors who trained as psychiatrists – Patte Randal and Josephine Stanton – and describes their journeys through the profession and as human beings navigating the vicissitudes, challenges, and traumas of life. Crucially, one of the women, Patte, has experienced psychosis herself and through that experience has come to see it as a spiritual emergency, a view that contrasts starkly with the medical reductionist approach of many of her colleagues in mainstream psychiatry. This perspective has enabled her to develop a more human and holistic way of approaching people who are experiencing a psychotic crisis. Readers will appreciate this book's openness and honesty. It testifies to the importance of being with and learning from people who have lived experience of mental illness and offers an uplifting, positive vision of the way that psychiatry can be practiced in the future'.

Richard P Bentall, Professor of Psychology; Author of Madness Explained: Psychosis and Human Nature *and* Doctoring the Mind: Why Psychiatric Treatments Fail experiences can share the significant value of their work. Complemented by international and national conferences and publication of the journal *Psychosis*, this series is central to the activities of ISPS and their global reach. It comprises books with a variety of empirical focuses and with differing experiential and disciplinary perspectives. Although diverse, the range of books combines intellectual rigour with accessibility to readers across the ISPS community. We aim for the series to be a resource for mental health professionals, for those developing and implementing policy, for academics in the social and clinical sciences, and for people whose interest in psychosis stems from personal or family experience.

To support its aim of advancing scholarship in an inclusive and interdisciplinary way, the series benefits from the advice of an editorial board whose members are drawn from across the ISPS community:

Katherine Berry; Sandra Bucci; Marc Calmeyn; Caroline Cupitt; Stephanie Ewart; Pamela Fuller; Jim Geekie; Olympia Gianfrancesco; Lee Gunn; Kelley Irmen; Sumeet Jain; Nev Jones; David Kennard; Eleanor Longden; Tanya Luhrmann; Brian Martindale; Andrew Moskowitz; Michael O'Loughlin; Jim van Os; David Shiers.

For more information about ISPS, email isps@isps.org or visit our website, www.isps.org.

For more information about the journal *Psychosis* visit www.isps.org/index.php/publications/journal

THE RECOVERY OF THE SELF IN PSYCHOSIS
Contributions from Metacognitive and Mentalization Based Oriented
Psychotherapy
Ilanit Hasson-Ohayon and Paul H. Lysaker

OPEN DIALOGUE FOR PSYCHOSIS
Organising Mental Health Services to Prioritise Dialogue,
Relationship and Meaning
Nick Putman and Brian Martindale

FINDING HOPE IN THE LIVED EXPERIENCE OF PSYCHOSIS
Reflections on Trauma, Use of Power and Re-visioning Psychiatry
Patte Randal and Josephine Stanton

For more information about this series, please visit: www.routledge.com/
The-International-Society-for-Psychological-and-Social-Approaches-to-
Psychosis/book-series/SE0734

FINDING HOPE IN THE LIVED EXPERIENCE OF PSYCHOSIS

Reflections on Trauma, Use of Power and Re-visioning Psychiatry

Patte Randal and Josephine Stanton

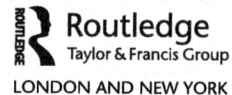

Routledge
Taylor & Francis Group

LONDON AND NEW YORK

Cover image: The 'It's About Time' hourglass design includes photos of Patte
and Josephine from childhood to now, crafted by finelinecreative

First published 2022
by Routledge
4 Park Square, Milton Park, Abingdon, Oxon OX14 4RN

and by Routledge
605 Third Avenue, New York, NY 10158

Routledge is an imprint of the Taylor & Francis Group, an informa business

British Library Cataloguing-in-Publication Data
A catalogue record for this book is available from the British Library

Library of Congress Cataloging-in-Publication Data
A catalog record has been requested for this book

ISBN: 978-0-367-72192-3 (hbk)
ISBN: 978-0-367-72190-9 (pbk)
ISBN: 978-1-00-315378-8 (ebk)

DOI: 10.4324/9781003153788

Typeset in Times New Roman
by Newgen Publishing UK

CONTENTS

CONTENTS

CONTENTS

ACKNOWLEDGEMENTS

As we began writing our acknowledgements, we wanted to include almost everyone we have ever known for the roles they have played in our lives; our families and friends, the people we have served, the people we have worked with, learned from, taught, the people who have talked to us and listened to us, the people who have not. The process of writing this book has brought out for us the significance of so many interpersonal experiences, some we might have thought unimportant or even wished had not happened. In the spirit of each crisis being an opportunity and the idea that what doesn't kill you makes you stronger, there has been richness in all of them.

We decided to restrict personal acknowledgements to addressing the specific process of writing the book. It has been a journey of several years and there are too many people to name individually. We proceed with trepidation because of the certainty that we will miss someone, and we hope everyone who has supported this venture will know our intention to include you. Thank you all.

We want to thank each person who participated in our research and who we cannot name. You have had a particular role in the development of this book. The richness in the stories you shared so generously with us was what got us going. Everyone who participated in our Sunday afternoon writing group took us seriously and encouraged us. Special acknowledgement goes to Kath Courtenay and Lil Ng for helping us to figure out how to talk with each other about the hard stuff. They are included in a long list of people who read part or all of the manuscript in its many forms and gave us feedback. Some of the people who read our drafts in the early days may barely recognise the final version. Your feedback has been vital in the evolution of the book. We have described duo-ethnography but there has been a level of poly-ethnography. Emotional responses, intellectually analytic responses, comments on writing technique, throw-away comments, questions, hard-hitting criticism, misunderstandings, and a sense of resonance with what we have been trying to do have all helped us get outside our internal experience and consider how what we are saying might be read and understood. Each contribution has been a practical lesson in holding the reader in mind. People in this list, in no particular order, include Tania Windelborn, Malcolm Stewart, Tony O'Brien, Jane Admore, Andrea-Rose McGregor, Debbie Antcliff, Sandy Simpson, participants in the Tauhara Women's Writing Away retreats, Nick Argyle, Lesley Mackay, Ann Pearl, Bruce Arroll, Christine Reynolds, Violet Sherwood, Dyana Wells, Tim Heath, Pat McGorry, Deb Heath, Jenny Heller, and Nikki Barrett. Many of our family members also read various drafts of the manuscripts and their doing that, and the responses they have made, have been very important to us.

Our ISPS editors, Anna Lavis and Andrew Shepherd, have found time to read and re-read what we sent in the context of endless Covid lockdowns in England and continued to work with us. They encouraged us and also gave us formative feedback. Though not always initially welcomed by us, we were able to work through a process where we felt that addressing the issues that they raised improved the book. We are too grateful to Susannah Frearson and Alexis O'Brien from Routledge, who welcomed our enquiries and supported the emergence of the finished product. We thank their reviewers who made valuable suggestions that helped shape what we wrote. Judith White also provided vital editorial input. She was able to grasp the essence of what we were trying to achieve with the book. She made important suggestions and questioned us about our writing in such a way that we felt held, understood, and valued at the same time as we were realising we needed to do some things differently. We also want to thank Tony Hadlow and the team at finelinecreative for the care they have taken and creativity in the cover and illustrations. In addition we would like to thank Dr Laurence Errington for doing the index.

It is also important for us to acknowledge each other. Writing the book has been a labour of love. Finding a way to contribute, particularly to the lives of people who experience extreme states, is dear to both our hearts. Throughout the process we have held one another in mind, and reaped rewards in terms of the way all our experiences have been validated. A life-enhancing bond has resulted from this sustained combined endeavour.

INTRODUCTION

I have jumped off the top of a flight of stairs, believing I would miraculously float to the ground as gravity no longer existed for me. I have travelled on the edge of time. I have been terrified that I, and my baby, were caught in a nuclear winter. I have lain on the floor of a mental health facility, believing that I could become two-dimensional and escape between the molecules of the wall.

I, Patte, am a doctor. The statements above detail some of my experiences. Psychiatrists would call them psychosis. Other people might say these are descriptions of 'mental illness', or madness. I call them extreme states. Because of my hope that my story will be useful to others, I have written and spoken about it publicly (Randal, 1999, 2012; Randal, Geekie, Lambrecht, & Taitimu, 2008).

On 14 October 2002, a doctor identified as having a 'mental illness' shot and killed Margaret Tobin, a senior psychiatrist in Australia (Sweet, 2009). Although such acts of violence are rare, when they happen they attract stigmatising publicity. Not only are they rare, but also people who are given the label of 'mental illness' are statistically much more likely to be a risk *to themselves*, or targeted *by others*, than to be dangerous. The publicity around this event could have increased any sense of stigma and discrimination I might have endured. In fact, this tragedy led, all these years later, to writing this book.

As part of their response to Margaret Tobin's death, the Royal Australian and New Zealand College of Psychiatry asked a team of psychiatrists to write about the needs of doctors 'impaired by mental illness' (Rosen et al., 2009; Wilson et al., 2009). Because of my lived experience, I was invited to be a member of this team. As I was starting to write my contribution, I showed an early draft to my friend and colleague, Josephine Stanton. Josephine commented on how she had heard me *speak* much more eloquently on the subject than I had captured in my academic writing. She suggested that perhaps it would be helpful if she interviewed me, and then the transcript of the interview could be used to bring to life what I was saying. As we did this

DOI: 10.4324/9781003153788-1

1

interview, we both realised the potential value of not only my story, but also the stories of other doctors who had lived through extreme experiences.

We undertook a formal qualitative research project and interviewed ten other doctors who had been patients of psychiatrists; five people who had, as life partners or friends, supported such doctors; and eight psychiatrists who had treated doctors as patients. Over the years of working with this data set, we have been increasingly struck by the relevance of the issues it highlights, not only for doctors, but also for everyone. We have published two papers in the open access version of the British Medical Journal (Stanton & Randal, 2010, 2016).

We were about to embark on two further papers. The first of these was about the way lived experience of extreme states impacts clinical work. Most of our participants felt that they had learned things that had enhanced their capacity to offer care in their doctor roles but had not found a way to share what they had learned. The final paper we wanted to write was about the way in which extreme states, including psychosis, were described by our participants as part of a spectrum of distressing experiences. There has been little published in the academic literature about extreme states such as psychosis in doctors, or indeed anyone in responsible professional roles. It is as if the world has been left to believe that these states do not happen to *us*, but only to *them* (those people who are not us!).

However, we did not feel our writing to date did justice to the richness of the material. It was hard to bring out the depth in the transcripts because protecting participants' privacy meant we could use only brief extracts from their full stories. Articles in the BMJ Open are available at no cost, but non-doctors are unlikely to read a medical journal. Writing for an academic journal also requires a particular style and approach which can be somewhat dry. Because of their general interest and applicability to everyone, we wanted to make our findings widely available.

I, Josephine, am also a doctor, a psychiatrist. Having worked and lived alongside Patte for over thirty years I have been profoundly affected by events which happened in her life and ways she has addressed them. In the context of our discussions of how to make what we had heard in the doctors' stories more available, I remembered enjoying the draft of an autobiographical novel Patte had written in 1989. A lot more had happened since then, but I realised that telling Patte's story, which we had permission to tell, could bring into the light all the issues raised by the doctors in our study and we had permission to tell it with all its richness. Patte's life demonstrates the occurrence of psychosis in a highly functioning person. We could show how the roots of psychosis were traceable back to Patte's childhood and influenced by her social and cultural heritage. Her story also exemplifies issues of power, gender, how pervasive are the effects of trauma, the importance of finding meaning in life, the need to find a way to acknowledge our vulnerability, the need for a paradigm shift in institutional psychiatry, the complexity of the doctor role, and the challenges in providing meaningful, healing relationships in a context of clinical care. The story is about psychosis, and many of us do not experience psychosis, but it is also about life, and psychosis is a part of life, an extreme part of life. It could happen to anyone under extreme enough circumstances (Mason et al., 2009).

Patte's development of an alternative approach to working constructively with people experiencing psychosis was informed and enriched at every step by her own lived experience. This mirrors what the doctors in our study described regarding the enrichment of their clinical practice and lives as a result of working through their suffering. Their learning could rarely be demonstrated publicly for fear of stigma and discrimination. Patte's story incorporates experience-based expertise, collaboration with the people she served, learning from experts, the courage and openness to think beyond existing models in terms of clinical practice and clinical relationships. Patte has packaged much of what she has learned and developed into a box, 'The Gift Box'. 'The Gift Box' is a resource that supports the development of self-understanding, self-responsibility, resilience, and well-being. It has evolved out of the work Patte has done over three decades, initially focussed on people experiencing psychosis but seems to be beneficial for a wide range of people, further demonstrating that understanding what we call psychosis has relevance to us all.

Finding a way to write the book has been challenging and we have tried many different forms. Patte had always wanted to include my story. Initially, I couldn't understand this but as we started to write, it became clear that my story could add a valuable triangulation as an example of another woman trained in medicine and psychiatry in the twentieth century. Patte's own story is an extraordinary one, with extreme experiences and extreme events; a story that must be told. My story is much less unusual but the essential issues with respect to contributing as a clinician to mental health care, and finding a way of living which has meaning, are the same. Including both stories is important because this is not a book about one extraordinary story; it is a book about issues that every mental health clinician – in fact, everyone – grapples with.

Our stories involve other people who have contributed in many ways to our lives. In the process of deciding who to name and where to use pseudonyms, we have tried to strike a balance between protecting privacy and making public acknowledgement of significant contributions people have made in our lives. Where possible we have gained permission from people we have named.

Evocative Duo-Ethnography: The Methodology We Used to Write This Book

In writing this book we wanted to use our stories to investigate wider social and political meanings. Auto-ethnography is an approach which seeks to describe and systematically analyse personal experience in order to understand cultural experience (Ellis, Adams, & Bochner, 2011). We have both grappled with the challenge of engaging in healing relationships with the people we serve. Our stories reflect cultures of medicine, psychiatry, the helping professions, and the wider society in which we live. In the process of writing this book, each of our stories became a lens we could look through to gain more understanding of this range of cultural and subcultural contexts (Chang, 2008).

In personal and professional contexts, we have both met and been influenced by many other people and ideas. We all bring our biases into research, whether they be overt or hidden. Telling both our stories has made explicit the contexts in which we each developed and lived. We also brought to this process what we had learned from years of reading and rereading the transcripts of our study participants. We resonated with them when they described their experience of mental health challenges as augmenting what they had to offer as clinicians, while not being valued in the system. The importance of lived experience and the perspective every one of us brings as 'experts on ourselves' are values we both share. Even without the study, we are far from neutral observers. Hope is important to both of us. We both work hard to find hope in all situations.

Patte's story provides the heart of the book. Initially the role of Josephine's story was to provide point and counterpoint. However, as we engaged in the process of writing we shifted our focus to duo-ethnography. This meant working together, each with an active role in writing our own and each other's stories and the meanings we have made of them as they have transformed over time. This process brought out a range of factors important in understanding human experience including trauma, power dynamics, the complexities of institutionalised subcultures such as medicine and psychiatry, and wider cultural influences such as gender. Exploring the extreme states Patte experienced provided particularly rich examples of the impact of these wider human issues.

Breault (2016) describes the intention of duo-ethnography being for two researchers to come together with their own current understandings of problematic issues. The researchers share their lived experiences in a repeated, reflexive, and reiterative process. They move to and from their stories, culture, and their different perspectives. Done effectively, this transforms their understanding. New dimensions of the issues will be uncovered and explored. This is the process we have used in writing this book.

Although growing up and qualifying as doctors on opposite sides of the globe, we both went on to train in psychiatry in New Zealand in the twentieth century. Our stories reflect many similarities to, and differences from, one another and our study participants. We were informed by our research data, our own lives, the cultures we live in, and our academic knowledge. Together we could examine our lived experience and training in psychiatry, while finding ways to be of service to people within and outside mental health care services. Together we could reflect on the lived experience of madness from the outside and the inside.

We were perfectly placed for this duo-ethnographic project. Over decades of friendship and years of being co-authors and co-researchers, we have built a high level of trust and mutual respect, which enables us to stay in a collaborative working relationship while questioning the meanings each of us has made of our experience. We have learned that our best insights come from times when our ideas and world views conflict. We need to stay with the conflict and work to understand both each other's and our own experiences, and emotional investment in holding our view. Then we are likely to move to a new level of understanding which takes us beyond our original stance. We understand this to be the heart of duo-ethnography.

Reading about duo-ethnography and making the process explicit enabled us to focus on the constructive potential of disrupting our own and each other's thinking. We developed an effective process of working together. In editing each paragraph, we learned to recognise moments when emotions were aroused as an opportunity for developing our thinking. We would slow the conversation, each notice our own response, name it and communicate this response to each other, rather than acting on it to defend our position. We then individually and collaboratively explored what underlay each of our views and emotional attachment to those views. As we did this, we were also able to bring in previous understandings, learnings from our study, knowledge of our culture, and academic literature in the area. This helped us uncover new dimensions of the issue and transform our own understandings, not only of ourselves but of the world we live in. This included the microcultures of medicine, psychiatry and engaging in clinical care, as well as the wider social context.

All our responses were worthy of examination. These might include a word that seemed awkward or unclear; a sense of lack of salience of a piece of writing; or feeling unsettled about what was being said. Words and phrases might attract questions and probing as to what the writer was intending these words to convey. Examples of these have included: intuition, truly, human, honest, 'so-called antipsychotic', patient, synchronicity, 'extreme state', client, 'people we serve', psychosis, mental illness, madness, religious, and spiritual.

Many of these words occurred much more frequently in the original drafts than they do now. We have chosen to use the term 'extreme states' interchangeably with the term 'psychosis', to emphasise the extreme nature of these altered states of consciousness. 'Madness' is a colloquial name for such states, which in the past had negative connotations but is now being politically reclaimed. 'Mental illness' is a widely used term, implying a biomedical model of pathology we are challenging in this book, as opposed to the social model of mental health and well-being that we and others are putting forward (Bentall, 2003; Moskowitz, Dorahy, & Schafer, 2019; Watson, 2019; Williams, 2012). We held a multiple focus with regard to how each of us understands the words we use, and how others use and understand them.

We interrogated any anecdotes which seemed long, wordy, or dense with information. An example that highlights this was Patte's initial description of the historical development of the ISPS (now known as the International Society for Psychological and Social Approaches to Psychosis). The account of dates, names, places, and events was not engaging. The discussion following this observation enabled Patte to investigate her experience of being part of ISPS over the years and how it helped transform her life both professionally and personally, an important case study of the potential contribution of alternative organisations. The results of this reflective process were often surprising and rewarding to us both. Effective reflection of this sort required acknowledgement, on both our parts, of the possibility that we each might assist the other in questioning and re-conceptualising our beliefs. We've needed to be willing to disrupt and challenge and to be disrupted and challenged. This process was at times painful. It needed to be supported by mutual nurturing and respect.

In writing the book we have used an evocative rather than an analytic approach (Bochner & Ellis, 2016; Ellis, 1997). We have chosen this methodology because of the 'abundant, concrete details' of personal, societal, and cultural issues it enables us to bring forward in such a way as to evoke 'flesh and blood emotions' in the reader (Bochner & Ellis, 2016). Through the process of writing and seeking feedback, we have often been surprised by some of the different ways people have identified with and related to our stories and the range of ways they describe being affected by them. Whatever analysis, reflection, and synthesis we make of them risks closing off possibilities of how others might engage with them. Rather than providing reflection and synthesis of the conclusions we have come to, we are telling our experiences with emotional presence to enable the reader to engage with our stories and make their own reflections and syntheses. We are hoping that as people read our stories they feel a connection with events in our lives and find something to enrich their own experiences.

Part 1

BECOMING OURSELVES

PATTE'S STORY 1951–1980 (BIRTH TO 29)

1

TRUST AND BETRAYAL
The Divided Self

In which Patte's experience of different forms of love, power and intimacy plant the seeds of later extreme states, and her life patterns of being superhuman and focusing on caring for others set the ground for induction into the culture of medicine.

It's 7 October 1945, almost six years before my birth. My imagination paints an unruly picture of the couple who are to become my parents. She's 18, curly black hair tied back off her freckled face, her arms around his chest as they sweep along the gravel road in dusty, parched Palestine. The handsome young man is 14 years older than his bride of three weeks. Their unborn baby, nestled between them, settles into the birth canal as the roar of the motorbike drowns out their laughter. Within hours this premature infant boy arrives.

My mother was born in Haifa in 1926, one of the first of the new generation of Jewish people living in what became the land of Israel. One of her grandfathers was a rabbi. Many of her extended family perished in the holocaust. Again, the history-making part of my mind flicks into hyperdrive. It's 1935. I see a little girl, nine years old. Her mother – my grandmother – has just died unexpectedly during surgery for the removal of her gallbladder. An open grave receives the limp body, wrapped in the customary white burial shroud. The child watches silently from her place beside her grief-stricken father. As the rabbi sings, she turns away, lost, alone; unable to cry. A thought crosses her mind. *Existence doesn't care about us.* This shattering idea takes up a central, guiding place. Even though she is still so young, my mother knows that she must become the author of her own life now. She must find her own way.

Her father soon remarried, but my mother never bonded with her stepmother. During my parents' wedding feast nine years later, instead of joining in the celebration of love and commitment, the stepmother insisted on 'sitting shiva' (the week-long mourning period in Judaism for first-degree relatives). We had always believed that this was because my father was a British policeman serving in the Palestine police force. He was the 'enemy' as far as Jewish settlers were concerned. The unearthing of our parents' long-concealed

DOI: 10.4324/9781003153788-4

marriage certificate recently exposed the 75-year-old secret of my brother's conception. We had all believed the wedding had taken place in 1944. At long last, what happened makes a lot more sense for a traditional Jewish family. Our mother had not only married a British policeman but also got pregnant out of wedlock. The effects of this secret reached through time, etching their imprint on my own as yet unconceived life.

Soon afterwards our parents and their baby boy left Palestine bound for England. A couple of years later my older sister came along. By this time, our father had gone to Burma to pursue his career as an engineer. Our mother, virtually alone in a foreign country, lived in a caravan with her two small children. At the age of 23, she and her two little ones eventually set off to join her husband. However, life had a different plan, as my older brother contracted polio. He would get better care and opportunities in England.

The young family arrived back in England in 1951. I can picture the scene. A ship berths at Liverpool docks in the early morning of an English summer. Sweet-smelling pink roses and pastel hollyhocks bloom somewhere in unfamiliar manicured gardens not far away. The foghorn blares. The sun breaks through the mist and warms the chill air. Tall and well built, my father manages two large, battered suitcases that have seen half the world and better days. A small boy with a calliper on his leg sits in a yellow pushchair, skilfully manoeuvred by an exotic-looking young woman. On her hip swings a cherub-faced toddler clinging tightly to her mother, afraid to let her go. The bulge of another baby is visible through the green linen dress. This was me.

What no one can see in my mother's youthful face is the grief of multiple losses. The loss of the two babies between me and my sister – one a miscarriage and one stillborn; the unresolved grief of the loss of her own mother when she was nine; and the loss of her dreams of becoming a lawyer, cut short by her first pregnancy. My mother's remaining family were all by now in Israel. Our father's mother had also died when he was a boy of seven, and he had left home as a teenager. In the intervening years, there was hardly any contact with his father, siblings, and stepmother. Despite this, my father's younger brother was there to greet them, bearded and hardly recognisable after all this time, doing his best to welcome his kin.

I was born later that year on 15 November at Mile End Hospital in London, under the sound of Bow Bells. Technically that makes me a 'true Cockney'. Actually, I never learned to speak Cockney. Our mother loved languages and her English was excellent, although she grew up speaking a mixture of Yiddish and Hebrew. Her intention was to teach us 'the Queen's English'. So, the way we spoke always differed from our neighbours in Harold Hill, Essex. Two younger brothers were subsequently born within three years of me. That meant there were seven of us living in a small three-bedroom council house, along with our father's various electrical motors and motorbike parts. Our parents slept in the sitting room.

Our mother always used to tell us that she and Daddy wanted to create their version of the 12 tribes of Israel, and to give us the opportunity to become 'free thinkers'. It turned out to be the six tribes of Essex instead, and we have since spread out with our own partners and offspring from one side of the globe to the other, but our parents did create a large vibrant family. We have remained deeply connected and loving towards one another over the past seven decades. Our father was a reserved, introverted man. Once back in England, he spent the rest of his working life as an engineer for Ford Motor Company in Dagenham. We children seemed to be mainly our mother's business. I don't know how active a role he had in this 'twelve tribes' idea, except that they seemed to keep making babies, which had to be partly his business too. How he felt about marrying her and having all us children, we can only guess at. Our impression, though, is that they always loved one another very much, despite their many differences. And, as parents, they were both utterly committed to us.

Our accents were not the only thing that set us apart. Although our mother did not practise the Jewish religion, she had imbibed the culture during her own growing up years in Haifa. Jewishness is handed on through the maternal line, and she saw us as 'the chosen people' – different and special. Although neither 'better' nor 'worse', this meant that we were not to consider ourselves to be like our neighbours. We were Jewish, whether we liked it or not.

I now know that losing a baby can affect the relationship between a mother and her next child (Markin, 2018). My mother had lost two babies before I was conceived. She told me that her family doctor prescribed vitamin E to protect this pregnancy. She was determined that I was going to thrive. She used to describe my early development in glowing terms, as if she believed she had created a superchild. She said that I was talking at six months; drew a picture of 'Daddy' at 18 months; and at three years announced that I'd been thinking about how people came to exist. Apparently, I figured out that my mummy's mummy must have given birth to her, and her mummy's mummy must have given birth to her mummy and so on, but the very first mummy must have grown out of the ground. I wonder now whether there was an element of idealisation of me in the context of her unresolved grief for the babies who died. Maybe it left me without much permission to be an ordinary little girl. My childhood memories are mainly of happy times. It is only in retrospect that I have understood the challenges I negotiated in my childhood.

With all her investment in me as this special superchild, she must have been beside herself when I developed asthma at six months after a cat slept on me when I was asleep outside in my pram. Often, my mother had to be awake at night trying to soothe me, and once or twice had to take me to the hospital for treatment, leaving my younger siblings at home. My asthma abated eventually, but as a young girl, I would often be unable to breathe, especially when anything exciting was happening. My breathing difficulties weren't helped by the fact that cigarette smoke was considered harmless, and both our parents smoked in those days.

One of my earliest memories is of all sorts of monsters under the bed. I regularly woke up screaming, until the family GP suggested I should sleep with my sister. Our mother would put us all to bed around six o'clock at night so that she could have some 'peace'. My sister and I grew close during these years.

My older sister was a compliant 'good' little girl, whereas I was much more demanding. There is a story about me crying fiercely because I couldn't have a little bottle of milk like she had when she started school. I always had strong feelings, and my mother hadn't had the benefit of more recent parenting ideas like validation and helping a child to self-soothe.

'Temper, temper, temper!!' she repeated on more than one occasion.

I also recall the stinging sensation of getting slapped around the legs when I was a bit older. One day I was smacked lightly on the cheek at the dinner table, for something I can't remember. Leaning my head to one side, I cried out, 'You've broken my neck!' I stayed in that position all afternoon. Gentle mocking followed. In my childish way, I was demonstrating that I needed a different sort of response from my parents.

Daddy, as we called him, never raised his voice. He was often silently hidden behind a newspaper. My mother energetically ran the family. It seemed to work pretty well most of the time, although a terrifying angry scene has survived in my memory as a reminder that things were not always in control for my over-stretched parents. Our mother was yelling at our father and threw a hot grill pan full of almost-cooked lamb chops across the room. This extreme behaviour only happened once, but I don't remember feelings being talked about, or con-flict being resolved openly between my parents. Despite the lack of this kind of modelling, I eventually learned to control my temper. Sucking my thumb was my preferred method of managing my emotions in those early days.

My two adorable younger brothers had arrived in close succession. Though only 17 months older than the middle one, it felt natural for me to take up a role as carer for them both. One afternoon, when I was not yet four years old, our mother put us all down for a nap. Waking up to discover we were alone in the house, I dressed the two tearful little boys and, carrying the one-year-old, took the other toddler by the hand and headed off down the street to find our mother. Maybe this tendency to take care of my little brothers was the begin-ning of forming the superhuman identity later to be expected of a doctor in the twentieth century. Our busy mother had popped next door to plan dinner with Betty, our neighbour, as they communally shared household tasks.

Having put the rituals and practices of Judaism behind her, our mother did her best to assimilate into the local culture and community. We celebrated Christmas each year with stockings filled with post-war treats such as pink sugar mice, oranges, and walnuts, but the closest we got to religion was that our father used to say, 'Good night, God bless', when we were tucked up in bed. A rare and special moment of closeness. For a short time, we were sent along to Sunday school. This came to a sudden end when I was found standing precariously on the windowsill saying: 'Please God make me die cos I want to go to Jesus'.

At five years old, I started 'infants' school. My thumb sucking had become almost continuous by this time. Bitter aloes had been applied to deter me, but to no avail. My thumb was corkscrew-shaped and my teeth were crooked, but there was no way my thumb was coming out of my mouth! My mother told me that children at school do not suck their thumbs and I would look very silly doing that in the classroom. The day I started school I stopped the thumb-sucking and never resumed, not even in bed at night. However, I cried every time any teacher as much as looked at me. I remember the overwhelming feeling of vulnerability. How I learned anything is a mystery to me.

One day a favourite teacher, a red-faced grey-haired Irish man, asked the class a question.

'What does "eggifullapie" mean?'

My hand shot up. The teacher asked me what I thought. A cold, clammy, sickening sense of shame filled me. I felt undone. I had no idea what it meant. Little did I realise that it was a made-up word with no meaning. I had pretended to know the answer in front of the class and been found out. At that moment, I decided that I must always know the *right* answer, and never make a mistake. This idea has taken a lot of unlearning.

When our mother became pregnant again, our parents moved to a bigger house. Our youngest brother was born shortly after we arrived at our new home. I remember the pleasure of seeing the tiny pink baby in my mother's arms, wrapped in his white shawl. As with all of us, he was breast-fed on demand, but quickly settled into some sort of routine that fitted into family life. My mother was occupied with him a lot of the time, so, in the pattern of being a superchild, I took it upon my seven-year-old self to keep my two younger brothers out of her way as much as possible.

The new house was built in a cul-de-sac that used to be the orchard of a manor house. The street was surrounded by the original high red brick wall that enclosed the orchard, and all the gardens had fruit trees. I used to climb the apple trees with my two younger brothers and regularly put the heel of my shoe through the hem of my hand-me-down dresses. The orchard was bounded by a wooded area. We three children thought of it as an exciting enchanted forest and spent many happy hours there after school and at weekends playing adventure games together, with me in charge of my little brothers. One day we caught a snake. We were convinced it was a viper, the only species of poisonous snake to slither across the British Isles. Much later, the realisation dawned that it must have been a slowworm but in our childish minds we were heroes who had narrowly escaped death. We proudly paraded our conquest in a glass jar for all to admire.

By now, I was growing quite tall and skinny – my long, thin arms and legs often bare despite the cool summer weather. My toothy smiles were self-consciously hidden behind my hand. With a colourful ribbon tied around my neck, and a pink rose picked from a neighbour's garden behind my ear, my walk to school was always an adventure. A pretty girl friend invited me to her house one afternoon. There she was, in her bright cotton frock, sitting happily on her father's lap. My own typically Victorian father was a remote figure in my life. Although he always brought sherbet lemons and toffee bonbons home from work on Friday nights as a family treat, I could not imagine sitting on his lap.

At around that age, I began to steal sweets from the shops when my younger brothers and I were allowed to go on our own to spend our sixpence weekly pocket money. One day I noticed a shop assistant pointing at me. Shortly after this, my brother began to tell our mother what I had done. Before he could say more, I stopped him. I went into a rage and kicked him, accusing him of telling lies about me. Was it fury at his betrayal? Was it shame or guilt? I could not bear the thought of my mother knowing. Was it my fear of failing to live up to her shiny image of me? To my relief, she never questioned me about this misdeed. But that didn't help over the next couple of years as I lay in bed, listening for a knock at the front door. Terrified, I imagined that one day the police would be coming to arrest me.

Gradually I developed strategies to help manage these fears. I decided never to steal things again and always to tell the truth. A habit of shallow breathing made it easier not to cry so much. I think a lot of children do this as a way of managing vulnerable feelings. The problem was, I think it eventually made me forget how to cry at all!

In my eighth year, my mother realised I was short-sighted, and I got spectacles. Being able to see transformed my school experience. I won a handwriting competition. I started to enjoy the hours I spent at school much more and ended up doing extra activities outside the classroom, as I'd finished most of the tasks well before schedule. My teachers gave me the space to be creative – writing plays and painting pictures.

When I was about nine or ten, my mother organised for me to look after a little boy, Paul, who lived along the road where I walked to school. Paul had Down syndrome. I loved playing with him while his mother caught up with household chores. It was a year or so after this that I recall being on a train. I was fascinated by a small child sitting opposite me in the carriage. As the train moved, she was waving her fingers rhythmically in front of her eyes and appeared transfixed by this experience. I recall thinking that if we could understand this child and why she was behaving in this way, we would understand what it means to be human. I decided at that moment that I wanted to be a doctor when I grew up.

During the summer holidays that year, I went to stay with a close childhood friend of my mother, and her husband and two young sons. They had recently arrived to live in England. The husband was moderately well-known. In order to protect his family, I have changed the details of his identity.

During my stay with them, he was extremely loving and warm towards me, lavishing me with presents. He bought me a beautiful orange and green swimming costume. As one of six children, in a household without much money or fatherly attention to spare, this was a captivating experience for me. He had long golden curly hair and his red beard made him look very handsome in my young eyes. His broken English and foreign accent sounded exotic. In my 11-year-old way, I fell in love with him. He played his guitar and sang the folk songs that he had written, encouraging me to sing along with him, and praising me for my voice. I could become a folk singer too one day, he crooned. Gradually he began to touch me, hugging me tightly, and putting his tongue in my ear.

'I love you; I love you', he whispered.

Kissing me deeply, he would thrust his tongue into the back of my mouth. Beside me on the couch, his arm around my shoulders, his fingers would play gently with my barely pubescent breasts. When I was in bed, he lay on top of me. Somehow, his wife was never around.

I remained silent and still during all these encounters, not finding them frightening or unpleasant but feeling overwhelmed by the unbidden sense of excitement. The whole situation was beyond my control. A sense of longing and desire for this man arose in me. He was around 37 at the time and his wife was pregnant with their third child.

When I got home from this holiday, I didn't tell anyone what had happened. I missed him and wanted to see him. The next holiday I was invited again. The same things happened. Confusion and disquiet unsettled me. This time, on my return home, I tried to tell our mother that her best friend's husband had kissed me and touched me.

'He's an artistic, creative song-writer and people like that behave in unusual ways. Don't worry about it', she told me.

The sense of confusion deepened.

After he had a heart attack a couple of years later, he wrote me a loving letter scrawled from his hospital bed on fine expensive paper. Maybe he didn't expect to survive but he pulled through. I was in love with this man for many years, but I also hated him at times.

I did speak with the man years later. After my first 'psychotic' episode, the extreme state that emerged when I was 24, I 'knew' on some vague and unformed level that what had happened when I was 11 was somehow linked with these later experiences. I found a way to contact him from Brighton, where I was living by then. He came immediately and took me out to an expensive restaurant. Over a glass of white wine, I asked him if what I remembered from my childhood had really happened.

'Yes', he said, and indeed proclaimed that he had always loved me, that I was 'a very passionate young woman' and that he still loved me. If it weren't for his circumstances, he told me, he would have considered going away with me to make a life together. I didn't know how to respond. He was very successful by this time and had an international reputation. It is only in retro-spect that I have come to see that my own needs had never been considered in his scenario, neither when I was a child nor when I was a university student. He somehow felt entitled to impose his 'love' on me as if he believed it was a gift, when in so many ways it was a time bomb.

The topic of what happened was never mentioned again to my mother until I broached it in my forties. I remember her alluding to things that had happened to her as a child but denying their impact or importance. I don't think my father knew about any of this. Despite all this, I always felt close to my mother. We shared an amiable companionship, even though she would often accuse me of being defensive.

'I know you better than you know yourself', she would say, enigmatically, in the next breath wondering aloud how I could be so intelligent and yet so 'emotionally immature'. It's odd how I can recall these snippets but can't recall what I was doing that provoked them. When I developed a form of eczema on my face that I would scratch and regularly make bleed, she took me to a specialist. The diagnosis was 'dermatitis artefacta' – a self-induced skin lesion. Even then, no one tried to find out what had happened to me.

My life both at home and at senior school was generally happy, as far as I recall, despite this early sexual awakening. Several of my school friends spoke of having sexual encounters with their fathers, family friends, or other older men. It seemed almost normal. We all laughed and fooled around together during break times. I enjoyed my school lessons and did well in all my subjects. In fact, my mother always reported back after parent-teacher meetings that each of my teachers thought that theirs was my favourite sub-ject! I had a natural talent for art and painting. Once, when I was around 12, I painted a picture of a mother and child connected in an almost womb-like embrace. They had only eyes with no other features, painted in green oil paint on canvas. A family friend asked to take the painting to America to assess whether my natural talent should be fostered. My parents allowed me a great deal of freedom to express myself through the medium of my art-work; I would often stay up all night painting. Notwithstanding the fact that I wanted to be a doctor, I decided that I would like to be a painter.

'You can always be a painter but unless you go to medical school, you won't be able to be a doctor', my mother said.

She saw doctors as worthy of the greatest respect. I could feel her pride in my aspirations, but I had the curious impression that none of my achievements actually was mine. They always seemed, rather, to be hers. She clearly had the talent and ability to achieve in her own right. She set up an intellectual dis-cussion group in the local community called 'The Thirty-seven Club', when she was 37, and appeared on 'The Brains Trust' television show after posing a question to Jacob Bronowski. My father managed to get hold of a cathode ray tube and created a receiving device so that we could proudly watch our mother on black and white 'TV'! When my youngest brother began school, she got a voluntary job in the local Citizen's Advice Bureau. She seemed to be in her element, assisting the poor and needy in various ways. During school holidays, she would take me with her to visit various people whom she was supporting. Some years later, she qualified as a social worker and eventually became a team leader. I felt immensely impressed by her and saw her as a role model advocating for those less fortunate than us.

Thinking about it now, I wonder whether her life-long investment in me as special left me feeling that it was not the real *me* who achieved. It was her version of me – the precocious child who talked at six months and had figured out the origin of human life by age three. This did not allow for the vulnerable parts of me to be embraced. I recall one day, many years later, on the verge of my second extreme state, thinking that if my mother really knew me, she would die. I wonder if the terror of my mother finding out about my shoplifting sweets had its root in this idea. I feel sad that, even as an adult, I was never able to have conversations with my mother about things like this. I always felt I needed to live up to her expectations for me and not to cause her undue concern. I wanted to affirm her belief in herself as having been an exemplary mother to us all. Since comparing notes as adults, my siblings and I have discovered that we each felt we needed to protect our mother from our vulnerability because we believed she would not cope with our pain.

I met my first boyfriend when I was 14. He was a university friend of my older brother and he was 19. My mother took me along to the GP and put me on the pill. There was no dialogue about this; just an expectation that I would be sexually active, and there was not to be an accidental baby. Now that I know about her presumably accidental teenage pregnancy, I realise she wanted to protect me from what had happened to her. Nowadays, a sexual relationship between a 19-year-old and a 14-year-old would be viewed as sexual abuse of a minor. It was never discussed with me. Things might have been different for me had I been given an opportunity to reflect on the choices that I was making, and those that were being made on my behalf. She had begun to insist that we siblings call her by her first name. It's as if she wanted us all to grow up and be her equals. In retrospect I can see that I was being allowed a degree of freedom to act in adult ways, when in fact I was a child. On the other hand, she was trying to protect me from the consequences of actions she was allowing me to take as if I were an adult.

Nevertheless, I managed to get nine 'O' levels with mainly A grades. I remember being terrified of getting answers wrong in exams, and being utterly unable to go back over subjects where I had made a mistake because of the shame I would feel in facing any academic errors – an echo of my five-year-old humiliation.

My second boyfriend was even older than my first one. I must have been 15 when we met. He was Venezuelan, and 22. We fell deeply in love. He ended up living with me, sharing my bedroom after my sister had left home. When he went back to Venezuela, I was heartbroken. Pining for him, I lost weight.

My older brother was encouraged to take me to a party. There I met Mark (not his real name). He was nine years my senior and had a doctorate in physics from Cambridge. Not immediately falling in love with him did not deter me because by then I surmised that being in love only led to pain and loss. I was 17. I decided to become his girlfriend and soon moved into his flat in London. A commute from there to Romford, Essex, enabled me to do my 'A' level studies.

I managed to get a place at the Middlesex Hospital Medical School. When I left school, I was presented with a prize for my achievements. I had chosen the book by RD Laing called *The Divided Self,* which had been first published in 1960, putting forward the challenging notion that people who developed what was called 'schizophrenia' did so because of disturbed family relationships, and that psychotic states were understandable. This choice seems very interesting now, looking back. Did I have some sort of premonition of what was to come?

Before I started medical school, Mark and I went off on a holiday to France with two of his friends. While we were away, I began to feel very sick. It turned out that I was pregnant, despite my attempts at contraception. When my mother found out she promptly arranged with an acquaintance of hers to organise a termination of pregnancy. No doubt she was thinking of my medical school education in the light of her own missed opportunity at a professional career. My mother's acquaintance knew of a private gynaecologist. All I had to do was get a letter from my family doctor in London. The family doctor was very kind. He tried to explain to me that this was a real baby I was about to kill and that I would regret it. I wrote him a long letter explaining that I respected his views but did not see things that way. I can see now that the views I was expressing were not my own, but my mother's. It's as if there was no separation between us. My identity was so bound up with her that I had no way of discerning what I really felt or thought about things.

The termination duly took place. I gave the gynaecologist an oil painting that I had painted, as a gift. It was of a very sad-looking young woman holding her hands over the place where her baby would have been. For many years I suffered silently for the loss of that baby. My mother never had any doubt that it was the right decision, but we never talked about it. I don't remember even discussing or reflecting on my feelings about the pregnancy and what having, or not having, the baby might mean to me. Maybe this was because my mother felt she had to keep the truth about her own unplanned pregnancy a secret from us all. In my inner world for several years following the termination of my pregnancy, the sound of *that baby crying* would often disturb me. Sometime later, after Mark and I had been married for three years and had another baby, I wondered what would have happened if we'd kept the first child. But of course, it was too late by then and we, too, never spoke about it. What comes to me as I write this is that maybe the crying that I heard was my own.

In writing this chapter for this book, I have been looking at my childhood thinking about where the roots of my extreme states might lie. But I enjoyed my childhood. Life at home was always very family oriented. I remember much hilarity at family meals on the weekend. My older brother would entertain us all with his rendition of Neddy Seagoon from *The Goon Show*, and my sister and I would have great fun dancing together in our matching crimson blouses at the local youth group disco. During school holidays, at four o'clock in the morning, our father would pile us all into the big old Humber-Super-Snipe car, our mother by his side, and take us on long day trips to Sherwood forest, Clacton, or even further afield. He had a sense of adventure.

Until I was around 50, my memories of growing up were of happy family times. It was only then that I became aware that life had been more painful than I had allowed myself to know. As for my mother, and the doctor culture I was about to enter, avoiding awareness of vulnerability was a central survival strategy. It worked, but only up to a point. The downside for me was that it left me open to the emergence of extreme states. It is only since I have learned to embrace my own vulnerability that I have become more resilient – but that's the story that will be told in the following chapters.

2

MEDICAL SCHOOL

Skeletons, Cadavers, Gray's Anatomy, and Desensitisation

In which Patte enters the microculture of medicine and begins to take on the doctor identity, further exploring love, power and vulnerability in personal and professional relationships.

Going to medical school in 1969 was an amazing experience. I was one of 18 girls in a class of 84. Unlike me, many of the others were from medical families and had been to elite fee-paying schools. We were mainly aged 18 or 19. I always sat at the front of the lecture theatre and quickly made friends with a young man who was slightly older and had been to Eton. His father was a Harley Street specialist. He became my physiology partner. We would always pair up in the practical classes to learn how to take one another's pulse or blood pressure, and work out our lung capacity and blood gases and such like. It was enormous fun.

I loved medical school and attended every single lecture. Each day I would dress in my smart, burnt-sienna-coloured suit with seventies' style wide shoulders and a plaid skirt cut on the bias. I'd then put on my high heeled shoes. The commute on the London Underground from where I lived with Mark took around 30 minutes. I would walk from the tube station to the Middlesex Hospital Medical School, which was situated behind Oxford Street, close to the newly built Post Office Tower. At the time this was the tallest building in London. Having grown up in the suburbs, being in the city felt very special – exhilarating. We were becoming doctors! There was nothing in the world more important to me. I was thrilled by the sense of privilege and honour.

From the beginning, our lecturers made it clear that being a doctor was not like any other career. We were to become completely trustworthy in our profession. People were going to look up to us. We must be entirely worthy of their respect and trust. We were to become doctors and be doctors in every aspect of our lives. Even on Saturdays and Sundays we were to be doctors, whether on or off duty. If someone collapsed in front of us while we were out shopping, for example, we were to respond as doctors. We were no longer 'the

DOI: 10.4324/9781003153788-5

general public'. We were going to be totally knowledgeable in our subject. There was no room for mistakes. So, we were to exchange our ordinary mortal identities for the superlatively rarefied identities of the medical fraternity. We were to become superhuman. The consultants in the hospital across the road from the medical school seemed like gods to us (and certainly to my mother!) As I reflect on this description now, the messages we were given about the power and authority to be invested in us are writ large. No wonder I had such a sense of awe and responsibility at the prospect of joining the ranks. It seemed almost unattainable for me, coming from such humble beginnings.

One weekend, I was sitting in the passenger seat beside Mark as we drove up North on the M1, Britain's first motorway, to visit his parents. It was pouring with rain. We were both wearing brand new, pale blue woollen sweaters. Suddenly the cars in front of us slowed down. Several skidded. With a shriek of tyres and a loud bang, the car immediately ahead of us crashed into the car in front of it. Mark carefully slowed and stopped. Without a word I leapt out of the car and rushed to the stricken driver, who had clearly hit his head on the windscreen and was bleeding profusely. This was before the days of compulsory seat belts. The fact that my medical school education had in no way equipped me to deal with this real-life emergency eluded me as my budding illusion of super-humanness came to the fore. I grabbed the door handle and pulled open the door.

'Don't worry! I'm a medical student!'

I don't remember what happened next except I know my new pale blue sweater became spattered with blood. I had no idea what to do.

On the first day of our human anatomy classes, I trooped into the anteroom of the anatomy hall with my fellow students, in allocated groups of six. Before we entered the hall, the pungent and overwhelming smell and eye-stinging sensation of formaldehyde assaulted our senses. The second assault to our eyes as we were led into the enormous hall was the sight of row upon row of metal tables on which lay the naked, grey cadavers that we were to spend the next term dissecting.

Our anatomy tutor had told us in hushed whispers that these cadavers had been generously donated to medical science. Our three-hour, twice-weekly dissection sessions were conducted in respectful semi-silence. We were instructed almost reverently to uphold the dignity of our subject matter at all times and to treat this whole endeavour with the utmost confidentiality. At no stage were we given the opportunity to reflect openly on the fact that these were the bodies of people who had recently been living fathers, mothers, brothers, sisters, sons, and daughters. The absolute mess we made of the no-longer human bodies before us was never discussed or acknowledged in any formal way. I understand that, in at least some medical schools, things have changed. But for us it was almost as if these were dehumanised objects, just as we were to become gradually dehumanised as we took to them with our scalpels.

23

We stood around our designated table in a pattern that remained the same from week to week: one person on each leg; one on each arm; one on either side of the abdomen. We were somehow meant to know how to dissect out the layers of skin and fascia, revealing all the muscles, nerves and underlying structures. I felt sick and a bit overwhelmed those first few times we congregated there, but I didn't say anything and no one else did either. It was hard to get rid of the smell of formaldehyde. Gradually I became desensitised.

There were stories of black humour expressed over glasses of beer in the common room in the evenings. I guess others found their own ways of releasing the tension, but I was never there. I went back to the flat with Mark and never mentioned my dissection classes until the very last week of the term. It was time to dissect the head. To my utter horror, I found that we were expected, literally, to saw the head in half in order to peer inside and dissect the brain. I couldn't restrain myself after this. To me it was an unbelievable atrocity in the name of learning. I told Mark all about it. He never really forgave me. Somehow, I had forever spoiled his shiny impression of doctors. It was downhill from there.

At home with Mark back in 1970's London, it became almost a joke that becoming a doctor involved macabre rituals and practices. At medical school, however, it was all deadly serious. There was no room for human emotion such as the natural distress humans have when initially encountering death. The fact that it was never talked about was a practical lesson early in our training in avoiding awareness of our own vulnerability. Doctors were somehow above and beyond all that.

Like a frog heating up in water and so acclimatising to the temperature that it does not jump out even at boiling point, I too was being affected by a potentially irreversible process. It's as if we were systematically being desensitised so that the normal human emotions of distress, anxiety, grief, and pain would no longer affect us. We were developing the superhuman capacities of our rightfully esteemed profession. Although there were unquestionable benefits of being part of the fraternity of medicine, I risked shame if I fell short of the expected ideal. There was limited room either at medical school or at home for the authentic, vulnerable part of me that might once have cried or expressed anger. My childhood pattern of shallow breathing to suppress emotion became an essential survival strategy in my evolution as a doctor.

Another aspect of learning anatomy was the imperative to own a skeleton. I inherited one from an Indian doctor my parents knew. Occasionally he and my father used to drink whiskey together. When I was accepted as a medical student, my parents' friend had proudly presented me with his very own copy of Gray's Anatomy, the one that he had used as a medical student himself, published in 1932. The doctor had inscribed in his barely legible handwriting in the already ancient anatomy book, which I still have in my possession:

To Dear Pat (sic)

The best of luck for your future & just remember this (apart from a few changes) is one of the two fundamentals of your future knowledge as a doctor.

With love

If only I knew what the second of the two fundamentals of my future knowledge as a doctor was meant to be!

He also proffered an old wooden box that contained a real human skeleton. No one was sure where this had originally come from but on more than one occasion it accompanied me on the underground to medical school, heavily disguised as an old wooden box.

Somehow or other, despite the aforementioned challenges, I was able to learn anatomy. I loved learning physiology, biochemistry, and pre-med pharmacology and seemed to have no difficulty committing the facts to memory. However, I do remember that revising for the exams at the end of the 18 months of my pre-med course was almost impossible. I would sit down with my books and wake up an hour or two later having fallen asleep mid-sentence within a few minutes of trying to focus. This happened repeatedly.

During this time, Mark moved to Sussex to take up a position at the university there. We had become used to one another's company and enjoyed the banter of academic discussion. I once accompanied him to a conference in Europe, and I used to help him write his academic papers for publication. I had no official recognition but it felt exciting to me to be contributing to the academic literature in that way. Like many women I contributed freely to supporting my partner's career with no official recognition. During my medical school holidays, I even worked as his paid research assistant at the research unit in London where he was employed. He was developing mathematical models to assist with town planning. I helped him gather data about the quality of shopping centres in a London suburb by designing a way of evaluating the appeal of shop-front displays.

When Mark moved to Sussex, I moved into the student accommodation in London – spending part of my time staying with him and commuting to London; and part of my time in the hall of residence. I became very tired and disillusioned when he was unable or unwilling to return the attention in support of my studies that I was according him in his work. Fortunately, I passed the first part of my formal medical exams.

Then came the shift to the wards. Shadowing the on-call senior registrar, I watched him attend to a cardiac arrest. He put huge effort into trying to save the life of the man whose vital signs had suddenly flattened to straight lines on a monitor. Sirens brought the team hurrying to the bedside with the resuscitation trolley. There was a flurry of intense activity with the administration of cardiopulmonary resuscitation, but nevertheless the man died. I was simply

25

an onlooker, but I felt the enormous weight of responsibility bearing down on me as a young doctor-to-be. In a few short years, I would be expected to perform and take the lead in this potentially life-saving heroism. The idea terrified me.

After the curtains had been finally closed around this poor deceased man's bed, the senior medical registrar must have noticed that I was on the verge of tears. He indicated that I was to follow him, and he took me to his private room deep in the bowels of the hospital – somewhere I had never ventured previously. He was understanding, even compassionate, in directing me towards the way I should be acting now that I was a student doctor. Whatever he said helped calm my fears and also helped me to feel that I, too, mattered, not so much because I was human, but rather because I was now a member of the fraternity. He was so valiant and cool in the face of an emergency and he managed the inevitable loss of patients' lives with fortitude. At the same time, he demonstrated a willingness to support and acknowledge me as his young medical student. I felt that becoming a doctor was still worth aspiring to, despite the enormity of the task that lay ahead.

Students become doctors by a process of apprenticeship. We were expected to be fast learners and not require a lot of nurturing. This was ironically described as 'see one, do one, teach one'. The messages were subtle and sub-liminal and hard to identify in detail but this sequence of events, like many others in my training, conveyed to me the style and skill required in medical practice. It also conveyed that it was not appropriate or wise to need too much support or to be vulnerable as a doctor.

3

AN EXTREME STATE AND
A SENSE OF PATHWAY

In which Patte's meaning making and coping strategies are overwhelmed by a series of intense, unrelated changes and events and new possibilities emerge.

In contrast to this registrar's attention, Mark's nonchalant dismissal of my worries felt jarring and uncaring. It created an unbridgeable chasm between us. I decided not to return to Sussex for the time being but to stay in London with my medical student colleagues, and try my best to manage the clinical years on my own. A week later there was a knock at my door in the student's residence. It was Mark.

'All my girlfriends leave me. I don't want you to leave me. Will you marry me?'

Was this a romantic proposal or an attempt to avert the death throes of an unworkable relationship? I was never quite sure why I accepted, but I did. Within three weeks we were married in a registry office accompanied by both sets of parents, with me wearing a pretty white summer dress I had hurriedly bought in Brighton the day before. It was hardly a wedding. But soon we went off for six weeks on a surprisingly lovely honeymoon in Kenya and Tanzania, where Mark's brother was working as a teacher. We went on safari in the Serengeti, climbed Mount Kilimanjaro, and snorkelled over the most superb jewel-encrusted coral reef somewhere off the coast of Africa. It was like an impossibly happy dream. Could it conceivably last a lifetime?

Then Mark bought a beautiful little house in Lewes, Sussex, which we decorated with hessian wallpaper. I was now commuting daily to London in an attempt to continue my clinical training. At weekends we would host Mark's university friends to dinner parties, up to 12 of us sitting around the six-foot wooden table that he and I had made together. I remember making my own 21st birthday cake with a house full of smiling guests and family members, thinking that my life had truly changed. Did I dare hope that the chasm between us would gradually diminish? We were able to be very creative together when engaged in Mark's world doing what he enjoyed, making our own furniture and building a home. I wasn't sure about where my life plans

DOI: 10.4324/9781003153788-6

fitted in the picture, but I was prepared to participate in Mark's world as best I could. Maybe I was repeating the pattern laid down by the encounter with the man in my childhood, letting myself be swept along with his agenda.

The next summer, I accompanied him as his wife on another amazing trip, this time around America and Canada on Greyhound Buses. Mark had been invited to visit a dozen universities to present his research findings and discuss cutting-edge topics.

Back home, it seemed from the outside as if we were a good couple, but it became clear that commuting for an hour and a half on the train to London from Sussex each day as a medical student was not going to work. I needed to find a way to make my life fit into Mark's world. So, with the support of the dean of my medical school, I joined the second year of a brand new neuro-biology course at Sussex University with the plan that I would return to my clinical training after graduation.

It was an absolute joy to engage in the academic work of my degree. I found being in this university environment so much more stimulating than the rote-learning apprenticeship mode of medical school. I loved the lectures and the studying. Amongst a number of rich and varied tasks, I did a research study with baby mice to find out whether a group of genetically identical mice would develop more dendritic connections if they were raised in an enriched environment, compared with a second genetically identical group raised in a deprived environment. The nature versus nurture controversy was raging at that time and my results strongly supported the role of environmental influences. Looking back, it seems so obvious that what is important is not trying to prove whether nature trumps nurture, or vice versa, but how they interact. Current epigenetic research is exploring how environment can affect genes, and we now know that it can affect the expression of genes even in later generations. Neither side of the controversy predicted that. Who knows where all this will go in the future but in 1972, I felt as if I was on the cutting edge of science even as an undergraduate.

Another fascinating and absorbing project that I engaged in with enthu-siasm was a series of interviews with child actors who were spending their early lives performing in stage shows around London. I wanted to ascertain the impact of their experiences on their development and quality of life. I also interviewed their parents. I managed to recruit at least half a dozen young protégés.

Mark and I also began to enjoy a full social life with his researcher friends, going out to dinner, or movies in Brighton, or hiking adventures in the Peak District or the Lake District; also visiting our respective families of origin in Essex and the Midlands. Married life was becoming comfortably containing, if not, for me, the truly romantic in-love experience that seventies' movies portrayed as the ideal.

Ever since I could remember, I had longed to have a baby. Somehow the memory of the ungrieved for child we had aborted had hidden itself in the shadows of my imagination. I decided that it might be a good time to have a baby now that I was not at medical school. Mark agreed. I was due to be taking my final exams in the May of 1974 and did not expect to become pregnant quite so quickly. By the time I was sitting for my finals, I was just beginning to feel the first fluttering of our baby's movements. I was so excited. The exams passed in a whirl of fun as I began to plan for this already much-loved child to enter our lives. It was a bonus to find that I had graduated with first class honours. I was offered the opportunity to take up a doctoral position in the department of psychology. It was not a difficult decision. My return to medicine needed to wait in any case as my baby would now take priority. I was due to enrol for my doctorate on the same day that he was due to be born. In the event, he was two weeks late. They were the longest two weeks of my life.

Having a baby was utter bliss. My academic studies continued unabated. My little son came with me wherever I went in those first six months, sleeping under my desk at the university as I began to formulate my proposed doctoral research project. Mark and I incorporated him into our lives as if nothing had really changed. He accompanied us to all our usual social engagements. He fitted in and he thrived.

What didn't work so well for me was our marriage. I was unable to feel Mark's warmth and caring. Even to this day, I do not fully understand why I was unable to reciprocate. We tried going for counselling sessions with Dr Anthony Ryle (now internationally renowned for developing his own psychotherapy approach) at the University Health Service. Instead of getting closer to Mark, the unbridgeable chasm that I had always sensed between us continued to widen for me. By the time our baby was seven months, Mark had decided that I was too unhappy to remain with him. Without any real discussion, he loaded me and our little son into his car and took me back to my parents' place in Essex.

I never expected that this would be the end of our marriage. Although it's true that I was not happy in my relationship – as I did not know how to identify or communicate what I wanted or needed – actually I was delighted with my little boy and with my studies. But in fact, I never went back to live with Mark. He never came to get me. We just didn't know how to mend things. Somehow, though, we stayed in close contact and shared the care of our son. To this day we remain committed to him as his equally loving parents, and we are very proud of him.

Eight months after Mark's departure I suddenly became psychotic. I didn't know it was psychosis. For me it was a mystical experience, full of meaning and revelation. I was living with friends in Brighton and engaging in a new lifestyle as a single parent. I was 24 years old and trying to get my head around the Chinese philosophy of health because my doctoral thesis was about researching the practice of pulse diagnosis at the fulcrum of traditional acupuncture. This was a new subject in the context of seventies' academia, and to do it justice meant embracing and trying to understand something about Taoism, a whole new meaning-making perspective for me.

My father had died of lung cancer six weeks previously. He had smoked 60 cigarettes a day for decades. While I was staying with my parents, he had confided in me that he was coughing up blood. I guess because I had been a medical student, he felt he could tell me. He was a gentle, caring, and responsible father, as well as an exceptionally clever man and talented mathematician, but I had never felt close to him growing up. As a teenager I had spent endless uncomfortable minutes sitting next to him as he drove me to high school, every day for five years, saying nothing. Maybe he was just shy. He was born in 1911 at the end of the Victorian era when children were seen and not heard. I had never heard him speak openly about personal matters. Never did he talk about dying, not even to my mother.

He had been so proud of me when I graduated, by that stage almost nine months pregnant, in my homemade, black maternity dress, flowing black robes, and mortar board. I knew he was proud because he gave me a gift of 50 pounds to buy a pram for when the baby came. Despite my medical knowledge, I never even considered that he would die. He had taken redundancy and early retirement from his highly-skilled engineering job at Ford Motor Company, and he and my mother had been off on the trip of a lifetime, visiting all the European places they had not seen before. They had a wonderful time. I don't think I allowed myself to face the implications of what 'coughing up blood' meant.

I was in Brighton when I received the call from my mother telling me that things were really bad.

'Patte darling, please come quickly. The doctor says the cancer has reached Daddy's brain!'

Leaving our 14-month-old son with Mark, I hurriedly drove the 70 miles back to Essex. I was there for those last days of my father's life with my family, and I was by his side when he died. My father was 64 when I saw him take his final strangulated gasp. I never looked back to see the expression of peaceful relaxation on his face, which my family described to me later. All I could see in my mind's eye was the look of utter agony accompanying the last throes of death. That image was magnified when, in close succession, two babies who went to the crèche where my son was cared for at the university also suddenly died. In the midst of this shock-filled sequence, I found myself falling in love with one of my senior lecturers who had also been through a marriage breakup. He reciprocated physically but without relational commitment. At the time I had no awareness of the power imbalance and my vulnerability in this situation.

I was involved in an intellectual process of questioning my own world view and the meaning-making system of Chinese medicine in the context of my doctorate. The loss of my marriage and death of my father had been so closely followed by the cot deaths. I was engaged in a physically intimate relationship which crossed boundaries meant to keep us safe. This was on a background of the unprocessed losses, traumas, and boundary-violations of my past. How much it all affected me only became clear much later. Like my mother before me, I hardly cried or even acknowledged feeling any distress. In retrospect I presume those early childhood coping mechanisms re-activated themselves as they did in medical school – by holding my breath the tears were prevented from flowing. Little did I know that embracing vulnerability and allowing the tears of grief to flow is so necessary for healing to happen.

It all proved too much of an existential challenge for my sense of reality. It's as if the invisible anchors that held my world in place were being set adrift. Everything felt impossible to process. I continued with my studies and taking care of my little son, as always. I was fortunate to have the radical acceptance of my friends and their support in the shared house, especially with childcare when needed. I don't know whether they had any concerns about my behaviour in the weeks following my father's death, but I do remember some changes in my responses and behaviour that may have been early warning signs.

One evening, after a conflict-filled conversation with a visitor to the house, I experienced a physical sense of falling and then profound relief on feeling that my friend 'caught' me, holding me firmly in her arms and comforting me. I painted a life-size lime green figure leaping into the air on the wall of my bedroom. My friends appeared surprised. They asked me very kindly to return my room to its former state by painting over it in white when I was ready. One night I smoked one puff of marijuana for the first (and last) time.

Things began to unravel.

I am writing furiously; a stream of consciousness, trying to make sense of the meaning of life. I go to bed. I do not sleep.

Time stops. An eternal moment of terror.

There is a paradoxical, almost orgasmic ebbing and flowing of a sense of trust that seems to alternate with the fear, going on forever, and ever, and ever, culminating in an orgasmic, ecstatic climaxing of trust. A cosmic battle rages between trust and fear, and ultimately trust is the victor.

The whole of life reveals itself with such extraordinary clarity that I am utterly dazzled by the intensity of knowing. I must forget. I must forget the unbearable visions; I must forget the overwhelming sense of knowing too much; I must forget the unbearable pain and the anguish of seeing things as they really are.

A powerful, tangible sense of pathway pervades my consciousness. A knowing that my life has purpose and meaning. I am in the vanguard of a movement meant to transform those who come after us. I must impart what I know. 'Mind=Energy=Matter.' I have a clear apprehension that one day I will write a book called 'It's About Time', a book that will be a vehicle for this change process. I see an image of a bookshop filled with my book – its yellow cover gleaming, its title clear and bright for all to see.

31

After the eternal night: morning.

I know that I must burn all the notes I made the night before; ashes to ashes, dust to dust. Outside, in my pyjamas, I make a little bonfire and strike a match. Flames flicker and crackle as my erstwhile stream of consciousness disappears into the glowing red and golden embers.

I am now covered in smoky fragments of burned paper, in the bath with my baby son. He playfully pushes my head under the water. I am drowning. Sounds become distant and indistinct; there is pressure in my ears and my nose is submerged; is this amniotic fluid?

I am being reborn into a brave new world. I clearly see a vision of myself pulling people into this new reality.

My friends help me with my son that morning and take him to be with his father.

I am hitchhiking to the university and I know that everything has changed. Travelling on the edge of time. I am the Mother of the World. In this new world, gravity no longer exists.

I leap off the top step of a steep flight of concrete stairs.

Pain. My trouser legs are torn, and my shins are bleeding. Every bone in my body has shattered!! I am perplexed: what is happening? Below me I see a group of foreign male students walking past on the next level down. They call up to me.

'Are you OK?'

'No,' I call back. 'My legs are broken!'

The men shake their heads and begin to walk on. I know this is a sign that my legs have been miraculously healed. I jump up, seeing the men suddenly become magnificently God-like in appearance. I run down the next flight of steps to the path below and mingle with the students who are going to their lectures.

'We're all the same!' I shout, elated by the realization that we are all God-like creatures, beautiful and regal in our shape and form. I begin to hug people along the way, my face beaming. Some step aside in horror, while others hug me in return, spontaneously responding to my joy.

I run through the campus until I arrive at the student health centre, where Dr Anthony Ryle is the director. I dash down the corridor to his room and fling the door open.

'Why do you need to be here?' I demand of the bewildered young woman in his office. 'We're all the same!'

Tony Ryle stood up and calmly directed me back towards the door.

'We may be all the same but we're busy in here', he said, almost as if he was amused by my sudden inappropriate appearance. He was probably ten inches taller than me and twice my age, towering above me in his kind and affable manner. Gently he turned me round and pushed me back into the corridor. I must have wandered off at that time but later I was scooped up by my anxious friends and admitted into the student health centre under his care. They had beds there for sick students to lie on if they needed a rest during the day or maybe even so that they could stay overnight.

Insisting that I sleep on cushions on the floor, I made myself as comfortable as possible in this unexpected setting. I felt as if I were a child in a nursery. The following day I drew pictures of babies and children and of young people, adults, and old people. Perhaps I was exploring the whole lifecycle, trying to make sense of the deaths of my father and the babies at the crèche, the birth of my own baby, and where I fitted in the world.

One of the nurses who watched over me in the university sick bay eventually told me that I was behaving 'like a child'. Her tone was harsh and unkind. Actually, this response came as a helpful surprise to me. It made me realise that although *my* world had irreversibly changed, theirs had remained the same. It was incumbent upon me to follow their rules in order to be acceptable once again. I didn't look back. Within a few days I was recognisably my 'normal' self again. For the next five days I remained in the student health centre. My little son was safely in his father's care. Initially, it appeared that the medication Tony gave me had been very effective. Those pink pills may have facilitated essential sleep in the first two days but, unbeknown to the nursing staff and to Tony, I'd stopped taking the tablets after only a couple of days because they were making me feel so ill, with a dry mouth and nausea. I felt as if they were poisoning me. Instead of swallowing them, I hid all the remaining pills in a handkerchief and kept them as 'proof' that I had fully recovered. I did not believe I needed to be on medication. When I showed my little cache to Tony at the end of the week, he agreed not to prescribe any more for me.

Tony had given me chlorpromazine, a so-called antipsychotic medication. At this time in 1976 there were a few cases recorded in the pharmaceutical literature of extreme toxicity associated with this drug; an idiosyncratic allergic reaction causing cholestatic jaundice. In layman's terms, my liver was self-destructing and potentially I could have died. Although I only took the tablets for less than three days, two weeks later I became extremely sick physically. I was nauseated, with itchy yellow skin and the whites of my eyes turned bright yellow too. I needed to have a liver biopsy to confirm the diagnosis, which meant a stay in the specialist London hospital, lying flat on my back with my head tipped down to maintain my blood pressure. Not fun. This turn of events brought me back to earth with a bang and, if I had been elated or high before, I reached the lowest of lows as a result of this physical assault.

I returned to stay with my mother who was adjusting to the loss of my father. She did the best she could, but I remember her disbelief that I might have had a problem with my mental health. I recall her saying something about how her side of the family never had any difficulties of this sort.

I still did not cry or grieve, nor even really reflect on what had happened to me. I don't recall telling Tony Ryle about the man who had been inappropriately sexual with me when I was eleven, but, given that I later contacted him and met with him in Brighton once I was well, I must have had some awareness that what happened with him had some connection with my 'mystical experience'. I still did not realise the impact that those childhood experiences had wrought on my life and soul.

No one assisted me in understanding that extreme state. If Tony tried to do so in later weeks, I didn't have the capacity to understand him. In fact, I hardly understood anything he *said* to me in terms of his interpretations of what was happening to me. Perhaps the most important thing for me was the quality of his *being with* me. I felt I could tell him everything and had a *feeling* of being totally accepted, understood, and validated by him. I had a sense that he cared for me. I felt *held* by him. In retrospect, I recognised that Tony was being simply warmly present and listening to me. One day I even asked him if he loved me. 'In ways', he answered. But he also assured me that he had a 'gallery' of people who he loved 'in ways' as well.

I was forever trying to argue with him that in order to truly trust that I mattered to him, I needed him to see me outside his therapy room. I wanted some kind of romantic relationship with him. No doubt I idealised him and thought of him as the perfect partner for me, seeing no reason why this should not be possible. In retrospect, this seems outrageous but understandable. I suppose it was some sort of fantasy re-enactment of what had happened with the man from my childhood, and with my lecturer too. Tony was very clear with me that our relationship was contained within the room and could not go beyond there. This boundary caused me endless frustration, bewilderment, and disappointment.

Now I can see that one of the healing elements in the therapeutic relationship was that I could get angry overtly with Tony, which I never felt able to do with either of my parents for fear of hurting them. I began to express my angry feelings. I found that Tony was able to contain my hostility without rejecting me. He always used to tell me that initially I had seemed quite 'opaque' to him. Gradually I became more transparent. He said that when the time came, I would need to grieve. He was absolutely right but I did not understand what he meant.

One day, shortly before I became jaundiced, he did a home-visit because I was physically unwell, and he was worried about my little son and me. And once, several years later, after I graduated from Sussex with my doctorate and was back at medical school, I went back to visit him, turning up at his house unannounced. He very kindly allowed my son and me to stay the night in a spare room while he got on with his own business. Certainly, I had felt his agape love and that's what was so healing for me. I know his nurturing of me increased my sense of agency and resilience.

He was my very first teacher in the way psychiatry should be practised. What he demonstrated with me became the role model for what I did later in my own career in psychiatry. He managed the relationship in a quite different way from 'standard practice'. His boundaries were clear but not rigid. I did something similar many years later when I saw that the people I served were not getting better with 'treatment as usual'. For example, with some of the people who had been in my care as patients, I allowed the relationships to develop into more of a mentoring style of being with them. I found boundaried ways of spending time with them that strengthened the bonds of trust while allowing a level of healing that had been impossible within the confines of institutional care. These gradual, transformative practices were always undertaken in a considered way and within the context of supervision with senior psychiatrist colleagues. Eventually this approach gave rise to a research project where I was able to demonstrate its effectiveness (Randal, Simpson, & Laidlaw, 2003).

Even so, when I met Tony three decades later and told him what had happened in the interim, he was saddened. By then he was a world-recognised figure as the father of Cognitive Analytic Therapy, which had hardly been conceived when I first met him. I was giving lectures internationally about my research and the 'Re-covery Model' I had developed, and also speaking publicly about my story. I was proud of my achievements and expressed to Tony how much I had valued his input. I attributed much of my success to the foundation he had given me. Tony listened attentively as he always had.

'What I offered clearly wasn't sufficient though, was it?' he reflected wistfully. 'If it had been, you would not have gone through so many further episodes'.

I had never seen it in this way. His support had been life changing. He took the risk of treating me himself. He did not put me under the Mental Health Act and commit me to the local psychiatric hospital, although he would have been justified by the extremity and danger of my initial behaviour. Had I been locked in a psychiatric hospital back in 1976, when I was 24, what followed in the rest of my life would have been entirely different and indeed may have been tragic. Thank you, Tony (posthumously), for your wisdom, courage, and compassion.

Looking back, I understand my extreme experiences as metaphors containing images that are full of meaning for me. It is as if my life, or my outer and inner experience of reality, had become a cosmic battle between trust and fear; as if I was dying to an old identity and, passing through a moment in which I became the archetypal 'mother of the world', I was reborn to a truer version of myself.

Could I trust my *feelings* of falling in love with my lecturer? Was I to trust anything about the relationship with my ex-husband, the father of my son, after he had left me? Was I to trust what I was learning about the different worldview perspective of Taoism and/or the apparently solid foundation of the scientific method, which clearly had its limitations? Was I to trust Tony? My mother? The man who had declared he loved me as a child? Could I trust the terror caused by seeing my father's apparent dying torment? How was . I to trust life itself when it was clearly so fragile and unpredictable, allowing babies to die willy-nilly? On some deep level, it felt as if my whole world had changed, and if that was so, then why would I trust or believe that even gravity had stayed the same? Everything else had shifted on its axis; and yet somehow, trust had overcome fear and manifested itself in this seemingly 'mad' behaviour. In jumping off the steps, I was acting as if I would somehow float, unharmed, to the ground. Believing gravity no longer existed in my new world suggests that I no longer needed to be held down by the previous belief that I was fundamentally different from others. In this brave new reality, I could now see that we are all the same in some god-like way.

Out of this experience, an almost mystical sense of pathway emerged. It was as if life had a direction with a purpose I could find if I looked for it. On the other hand, at times I also had intense anxiety in unlikely situations. For example, for years after this first extreme-state episode, I felt intensely anxious when turning on the television for fear of what news of catastrophe I might encounter.

In retrospect, I can see that the real-life happenings prior to this extreme experience triggered a meaning-making crisis in my 'psyche' or soul. The hard reality is that gravity still existed, and it came back to meet me with a thump. The nurse's rather mean comments about me acting like a child were another example of the truly harsh world not having changed. Her uncompassionate response once again brought me into contact with the reality of human imperfection. It abruptly became clear to me, as if waking me up from a happy but deceptive dream, that I must take responsibility for myself in an adult way.

All the pieces of the jigsaw puzzle of life were plain to see, but at the time I was not ready to put that picture together on a feeling level. Somehow the psychosis protected me from the grief and sadness of it all. It got me through to the other side rather like being in a time capsule. Indeed, I clearly recall the sensation of travelling on the edge of time.

It is as if the experience of psychosis was itself like being confronted by a giant jigsaw puzzle, with the pieces strewn around for all to observe but with no clear picture to guide me to put the pieces meaningfully together. My world had been shaken up beyond recognition and I wonder now if the right sort of support would have enabled me to get to another level of self-understanding, which would have protected me from further extreme states as Tony had implied.

Many years later in a new country, with a new husband and two more children, I experienced another extreme-state episode. I had a clear vision.

I am completing a gigantic cosmic jigsaw puzzle. I feel overwhelmed by the enormity of what I have achieved.

A real-life juxtaposition of events followed. I came home from work to find that the children had tipped all their jigsaw puzzles on the ground and we were literally faced with the task of sorting out hundreds of pieces to make ten different puzzles. I remember the feeling of utter relief and satisfaction when all ten puzzles were complete. I also remember the intense sense of meaning that I experienced, as if one day I would indeed be able to put all the pieces of my life together and see what it all meant. I'm not sure that I have done that even now but, certainly as I write this 40 years later, a great deal more clarity has crystallised for me.

4

RESEARCH AND METAPHOR
Medical Nemesis

In which Patte explores contrasting ways of understanding the
world informed by lived experience as patient, budding doctor
and flourishing academic. She looks for ways of holding alternative views and stumbles upon biases in human thinking.

Within six or so weeks of the extreme state, and once the jaundice had
resolved, I was deemed mentally and physically well enough to return to my
doctoral studies without further medication. Neither I nor my family was told
of a diagnosis. I remained 'well', if rather anxious and at times unsettled emotionally, for around 12 years following this first episode.

I completed my doctoral studies in 1977. This was not only hard work
but also very stimulating. It opened my mind to a totally different way of
viewing health. I found from my reading of the Chinese philosophy of health
that I was developing a passionate interest in alternative views of healthcare.
Soon after recovering from my first extreme state/mystical experience, a friend
introduced me to the concept of 'synchronicity' or meaningful coincidence.
This friend also gave me a copy of the I Ching, or *Book of Changes*. It seemed
apt, given that I was immersing myself in Chinese philosophy, to embrace
this approach to life's challenges. At that point I began to play around with
asking questions of this ancient Chinese divinatory text by throwing coins in
a particular sequence. I guess I was searching for answers to what life had so
mysteriously presented to me.

I have some of the diaries in which I kept the details of my many questions
and what, at the time, seemed to be uncannily meaningful 'responses' from
that strange book. Some of these questions applied to my research journey;
some to my private life. I had the sense, however, that throughout my doctoral
years I was on some kind of quest to make sense of reality. Looking back
on those diary entries, I can see that my questions were often open-ended
and the 'answers' somewhat vague and open to multiple interpretations –
rather like a horoscope, or a Rorschach test. It all seems a bit like gobble-
dygook to me now, in 2020, especially with the I Ching's frequent references

DOI: 10.4324/9781003153788-7

to the 'superior man' and the 'inferior man', which, naïve to gender politics at the time, I took to mean aspects of myself. When I read those words now, I can't really even imagine what I made of them at the time. I had entered a new realm of seeking meaning beyond the everyday world, and had a frequent sense of life having a purpose and meaning beyond my own making. Even as I pursued the scientific method, with all its intellectual and practical rigour, the I Ching was my frequent go-to place for boosting that sense of pathway that had become part of my world following the mystically meaningful extreme state.

At the same time, I had a strong commitment to the scientific method. I also had an intuitive sense that the reductionist scientific analytic framework of Western medicine was limited in what it could contribute to health. I was excited by the idea that traditional acupuncturists were only paid when the people they served remained well. The entire purpose of the practice of pulse diagnosis and acupuncture was to help maintain the balance of 'chi' energy, or 'life' energy, and thus maintain wellness. If a person became unwell, it meant that the acupuncturist had fallen short of his or her function as a practitioner. I was fascinated by the fact that their beliefs were part of a different paradigm and worldview. I accepted this as being just as valid as the medical model and scientific paradigm in which I was being trained.

My research allowed me to encounter a group of people, all men as it happened, who were skilled practitioners in traditional acupuncture in England in the mid-1970s. Some had been practising for over a decade and had trained in China. They were the 'experts' in the field. Googling their names, 40 years later, has corroborated the recognition they received during their fruitful and contributory careers. Several were leaders who set up schools of acupuncture and helped bring credibility to their knowledge over the ensuing years until their deaths. One is still practising. It was an extraordinary privilege to work alongside them. In retrospect, I am humbled and in awe of the fact that they were prepared to put their skills 'on the line' during the experimental procedures that I, a mere medical student cum doctoral candidate aged 25, had devised.

I set up a series of experiments designed to evaluate the art of Chinese medicine using the scientific method. The acupuncturists believed they were able to reliably report specific pulse imbalances which correspond with particular diseases from pulse information alone.

As part of my research, I set up a situation where they, and a skilled anaesthetist as a control, were behind a screen wearing blindfolds and earphones so the 'patient' could not be seen or heard. The patients were wearing gloves and put their wrists through holes in the screen so that the only parts of the body that were available to the acupuncturist were their wrists. The only contact that the acupuncturists had was the tips of their fingers on the bare skin of the patients' wrists (see Figures 4.1 and 4.2). The patients had been chosen on the basis that they had severe pathology in specific organs (e.g., heart, lungs,

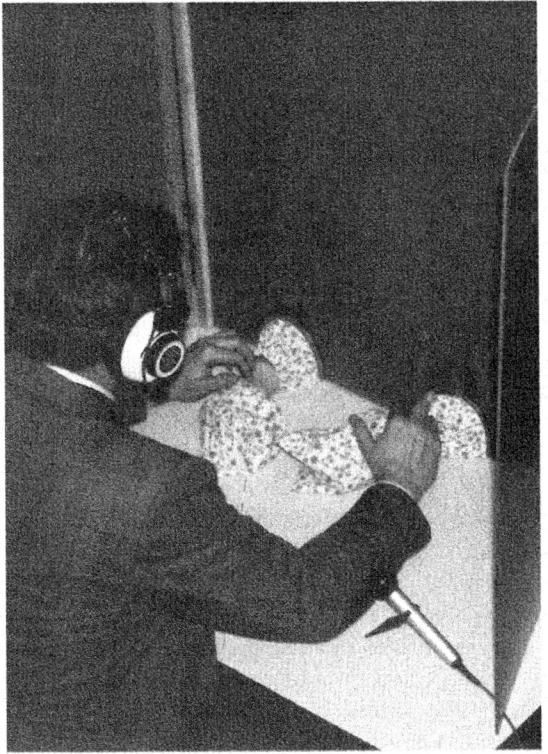

Figure 4.1 Photo of acupuncturist participating in pulse diagnosis research.

liver, or kidneys). Interspersed amongst them were healthy people without any known illness.

Although both the anaesthetist and the acupuncturists could distinguish those people with illness from the healthy people, none of them was able to identify specific organ pathology or diagnoses from pulse information alone.

In a very unscientific and human way, I felt shocked and disappointed at the results. I had believed and hoped that my research would validate the ancient practice of pulse diagnosis. The practitioners themselves were confident of their skills or they would not have participated in the research and I had no reason to doubt them. While I was becoming physically unwell after my extreme state, I had been to see one of the acupuncturists who was participating in my pulse diagnosis study. I was feeling extremely sick but had not yet become jaundiced so there was no indication of what the problem was. He took my 'pulses' in accordance with the traditional practice and told me I had a severe imbalance in my liver pulse. Several days later I turned yellow. This experience had a profound effect on me. I believed that the acupuncturists could do what they too believed they could do. I expected to find positive results.

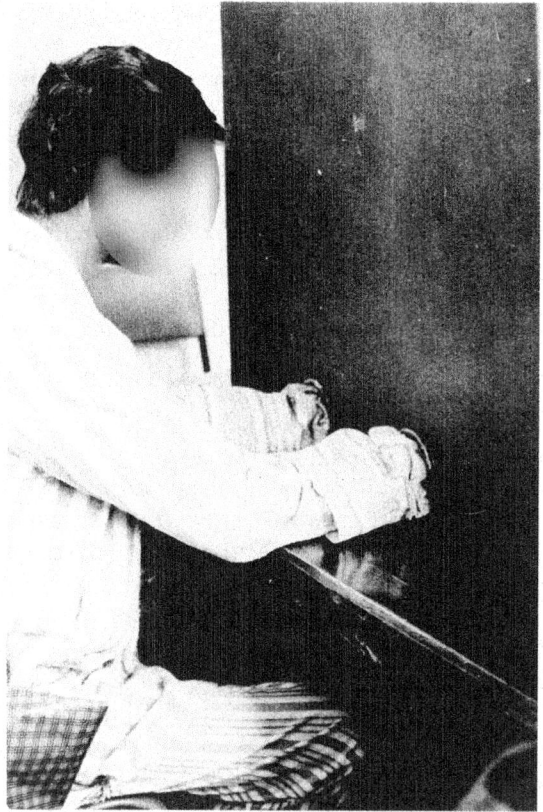

Figure 4.2 Photo of patient participating in pulse diagnosis research.

I found it hard to figure out what my findings really meant. What was hardest for me personally was that I realised that I had not devised a valid test of the acupuncturists' skills. The practice of traditional acupuncture was holistic. In 'real life', the acupuncturists would never be in this contrived situation. They had participated in the study in good faith. I felt I had let them down. This continues to be an important issue in research. Double blind randomised controlled pharmaceutical trials are seen as providing the strongest evidence for therapeutic efficacy, and yet they are routinely set up in contexts that do not accurately reflect the 'real world'. They have to involve people who can give informed consent, who are not on multiple medications, do not have too much risk or co-morbidity, and who usually will only be required to participate for six weeks before the results are evaluated. This very rarely reflects the 'real world' use of these medications. We are only just beginning to recognise the damage that such inadequate information has inflicted in the name of science. I was painfully aware of the inadequacy of my best attempts at applying science in the complex context of the practice of the pulse diagnosis. What could we really glean from my hard-won results?

I went on to develop a series of experiments using a simulation of the pulses and I generated a theory of why the skilled practitioners believed they could do something that my research proved was not the case. I had worked hard for three years, researching and writing up my thesis. My studies had taught me a great deal about how to do 'science': how to set up experiments, recruit participants, and analyse results. We usually think we know what is 'really' happening by everyday observation but, in the words of my doctoral supervisor: 'We can't "do" science in our heads'.

I had stumbled upon an example of the biases we all have in our thinking that result in our tendency to confirm our beliefs rather than refute them. It is obvious to me now that this is indeed why we need the scientific method. Perhaps most importantly I had begun to learn about thinking about thinking but I didn't realise this until much later.

What I was most interested in though were my attempts to understand and write about the Chinese philosophy of health. It was fascinating to me that the ancient Chinese culture that evolved the acupuncture system had never evolved the scientific method. In the first four chapters of my thesis, I put forward the thinking I had developed about the different approaches of Western analytical thinking and Chinese philosophical thought. This was the part of my thesis of which I was most proud.

I explored the differing focus of each way of thinking. I suggested that there is potential harm in the Western tradition of limiting the knowledge we value to 'analytical thinking'. I suggested that 'metaphorical' thinking of the Chinese tradition is the mode with which we attribute and experience meaning and value, enabling wise choices about health and wellbeing. I wondered whether its displacement by the seemingly superior analytical mode had led to severe problems in our ability in the West to apprehend the world in a healthy way.

I handed in my thesis and returned to London to complete my medical school training. Just before my medical school term began, I attended my final doctoral viva with Professor Patrick Wall (famed for the Wall/Melzack gating theory of pain) as my external examiner. I was dismayed to discover that I was required to rewrite the first chapter of my thesis and exclude the first four chapters of which I was so proud before they would award my degree.

Professor Wall commented, 'You wouldn't want your doctorate to be seen as your *intellectual autobiography*'.

At the time I didn't understand what he was talking about. It was as if he was mocking me. The first four chapters demonstrated the development of my ideas about the differences between the way the ancient Chinese made sense of the world, compared with the way people in the West think. The examiners were happy with my scientific findings but not happy with my exploration of what I called the 'metaphorical thinking' that underpinned the Chinese philosophy of health as opposed to the 'analytical thinking' that appeared to underpin Western academia. Although I can understand that what I wrote was truly a part of my intellectual development, I believe that it still has merit.

At the time, 40 years ago and for many years after, I felt that my research degree was only half what I had set out to achieve. Although I was able to complete the task of re-submitting my thesis during my first few weeks back at medical school, and I achieved my doctorate, it felt somewhat hollow. The piece of my work that I felt was of most value had been discarded. Furthermore, as I returned to medical school, my previously rose-tinted lenses that had enabled me to be so blindly positive about the experience of becoming a doctor, had been permanently discoloured. I had developed much more capacity for critical appraisal and an ability to evaluate the pros and cons of what medicine had to offer. I was able to stand outside the power dynamic of the culture.

5

COMPLETING MEDICAL SCHOOL
Examining Reflexes

In which Patte finds that the 'doctor-identity' has its surprising opportunities and dangers in terms of personal security and psychological safety.

On returning to London as a 26-year-old, divorced, single parent, medical student with my 3-year-old son and a doctorate, I was faced with various hurdles. First, I had to find an affordable place to live. This turned out not to be as hard as I was anticipating. I had a close friend who had helped me a great deal with setting up and executing the final experiments in my research. He was a doctor and he had contacts in North London who were in the squatting movement. At that time in London, housing was a political issue and a large number of intellectuals and professional people had taken steps to legally access empty houses and take up residency. My doctor friend found a squat for me in the basement of a four-storey house. It was spacious, dry and airy, and in a very pleasant area. I found all I needed to furnish it in the local second-hand furniture shops, which were full of cheap furniture largely from deceased estates. I remember faded brocade curtains that used to be Sherwood green. I lived there for about a year and survived at least one burglary without too much upheaval.

My second hurdle was finding childcare for my son. This too proved relatively straightforward. There was a highly recommended nursery school within walking distance of the medical school, which was prepared to accommodate him. He fitted in readily as he was used to being at day care. We enjoyed our trips on the bus to get there and back in the mornings and evenings, with me reading all sorts of books to him on the journey. The biggest problem was that the nursery didn't open until 8.30 am and children needed to be collected by 5 pm, and it was a half-hour walk to the medical school. My clinical pharmacology lectures began at 8.30 am, and my neuroanatomy lectures were from 4 to 5 pm. This meant that I was only able to attend half of every lecture for both courses. The faculty accepted this difficulty, but it did mean that I had to work doubly hard to try to catch up.

DOI: 10.4324/9781003153788-8

One Sunday, while travelling back to London on the train from Brighton on one of my trips to visit friends, I met a woman with a little girl of about my son's age. They sat next to me and we began to talk. She told me that her husband was away and that she was desperate to find somewhere to live in London. She seemed a pleasant and friendly person, maybe a little older than me, and her daughter was sweet. Given that I was living free of charge in a place that was not my own, and that there were two spare rooms, I gladly offered for her to move in. We discussed how we could be of mutual benefit to one another with babysitting and so on. Needless to say, she was extremely grateful.

Things seemed to be going well with this new situation for about three months or more. The children were mainly getting on well when they were together. On the whole, we were managing our lives quite separately but bene-fitting from the occasional opportunity to go out in the evenings as we were each willing to take care of both children when needed. Then one night around 2 am I was woken by loud banging on the front door; then raised voices and a commotion outside my room. It was the police. They had a warrant to search the building and arrest my new flatmate. I found out later that she had a printing press hidden in the shed at the bottom of the garden. Her partner was a member of an Irish anarchist terrorist group and was in prison. I subse-quently referred to her as an 'anarchist feminist terrorist'. I don't know what happened to either her or her daughter.

It seemed to me that I had made a serious mistake in inviting her into my home. As usual, I had been too trusting. The next day I made an appointment to talk with the dean of the medical school to ask whether my son and I could move into student accommodation as an emergency solution. The dean was concerned about my situation. After much thought and discussion with his colleagues, he made me an extraordinary offer. He was very apolo-getic that the medical school was unable to accept a child into their halls of residence but instead they offered me an interest-free loan to buy my own property in London. The loan was to be repaid once I qualified as a doctor and began earning money. Even to this day, it seems hard to believe that all this happened! The notion of the 'medical fraternity' took on new meaning for me that day.

I was able to buy a flat above a shop in Kingsland Road near Dalston Junction, London, where my son and I lived comfortably and safely for the following years as I continued with my clinical training. The flat cost 11,000 pounds, a thousand of which was provided by Mark and the rest was provided by the medical school loan.

It was 1978. Within a short time, I had found a delightful young live-in nanny, charming, funny, and fully trained in the art of childcare. My son and I instantly fell in love with her. Soon after, my sister, whose own son is a month older than mine, bought the identical upstairs flat. We were able to support one another as a family. The little cousins got on famously (and eventually went to school together) and we all happily shared our lovely nanny, who became like another member of the family.

Meanwhile my time as a clinical student 'on the wards', as we called it, was not only varied and exciting, but also daunting and unnerving. Being part of the 'firm', as the clinical teams were called, was always a remarkable experience, like walking on Mount Olympus amongst the Gods. We would trail around in our white coats with our stethoscopes around our necks, following behind our consultants, senior registrars, registrars, senior house officers, and house officers as they did their ward rounds, looking like a huge waddle of penguins with us juniors taking up the rear.

We armed ourselves with as much information as we could glean from our reading, or talking with the patients, or looking at their files, in case we were ever asked a question. Students were at risk of being targeted and publicly shamed in these ward rounds. Shortly after my return to the wards, I was directed by my consultant to 'examine the reflexes'. There was no mention of the person to whom these reflexes belonged and no asking the man's permission to take hold of his leg to perform the procedure. My heart sank. Despite being left-handed, I took up the requisite position on the right side of the patient's bed and held the reflex hammer in my right hand. The task was to lift the patient's bare knee and lightly tap below his kneecap to elicit the reflex. This is a muscle movement which would show whether his peripheral nerves were in good working order. Using my non-dominant hand, I tapped several times, producing a variable effect.

'That was disgusting', said the consultant as we left the bedside to resume the round.

In front of the whole team he told me that I should know how to elicit reflexes by now and that I would fail if I performed as atrociously in my exams. It seemed very unlikely to me at that moment that I would ever graduate as a doctor, let alone ascend to the shimmering heights of becoming a consultant.

During my time at Sussex, I had read a controversial book called *Medical Nemesis* by Ivan Illich (1975), which exposed power dynamics in modern medicine. He argued that the medical establishment had become a major threat to health by expropriating the power and control over personal well-being. This consultant's behaviour felt like a case example. He showed no interest in either me as his student or, more importantly, in the man sitting in the bed beside us. Any value or achievements I, or the man in the bed, might have had counted for nothing compared to the unassailably, bewilderingly unmatched wonderments of medical prowess, seniority, and superiority.

His belittling of me was an affront. It felt very unfair. A strong sense of justification at my lack of skill welled up in me. Given the long detour I had taken via Sussex University, with five years out of medicine, it was not surprising that I had some catching up to do. It did not mean that I would be unable to learn the skills of my chosen profession in due course. I decided that I was not going to allow him to hold a view of me which I considered so untrue and unfair.

I found myself at a collegial function a week or so later and this consultant was present. Approaching him boldly, I told him how glad I was to be able to be back at medical school after having my son and completing my doctorate. I told him that it was not easy for me being in this position. Remarkably, he was prepared to listen to my story and to acknowledge that given my unusual circumstances and my determination, I might indeed have a chance of completing my medical training. It was a relief to have had that opportunity to rectify his impression of me. After that, he was always much more respectful and supportive on ward rounds. I was glad to have the opportunity to stand up for myself. The man in the bed was not so fortunate.

Probably the strongest impression of my clinical years is the huge unearned privilege it always was to be in a position of trust with people as a medical student. To have people share their stories with me was always a pleasure even when the story was painful, as it almost always was in those circumstances. A medical interview was focused on eliciting symptoms and signs of illness with a view to deciphering what was physically wrong with a person. But it was still possible to hear the fascinating sequence of how individual lives had unfolded and to provide a listening ear in some cases where no one had ever listened to or heard these stories before. As a student it was possible to devote the time needed for this, even though it was not a designated task, and there was no teaching on *how* to listen effectively in a therapeutic way. Being taught about surgery was interesting too, but it took the form of standing for hours on end, gently holding the patient's guts wrapped in muslin, and watching as the surgeon cleared away cancerous tissues in the body cavity. Another level of human vulnerability was being exposed and it left me with deep respect for a skill I knew I would never choose to emulate.

I had a particularly special experience with a young woman from the West Indies. She had suffered a ruptured cerebral aneurism and was lying in a coma in a back ward of the neurology unit, needing total nursing care. She was breathing without life support and was being fed by a nasogastric tube. I decided to spend time every day sitting alongside this woman on the ward, holding her hand and talking to her, despite the fact that she could not respond. Perhaps I had an intuitive sense that on some level she was conscious of my presence and needed that human contact. This went on for several weeks while I was doing my student placement on that ward, with no visible improvement in her functioning. Even when I moved on to another ward at the end of the allocated time, there had been no change in her presentation. However, what seemed like a long time later, I went back to that ward to find out what had happened to this young woman. To my utter amazement, I was given the thrilling news that she had one day opened her eyes and started speaking, had regained full function and eventually left the unit. Was the time I spent with her useful? I will never know but it was hard not to hope that maybe, just maybe, the hours I spent being with her had somehow helped. Although far from the usual role of a doctor, this little mystery with a happy ending has remained with me all these years.

Eventually, the time came to take my final clinical exams. The written papers were relatively straightforward as I was so used to taking exams. However, although I had prepared as well as I possibly could for the clinical finals, I was so anxious about my practical viva that I literally vomited on my way there. Nevertheless, I managed to pass and at last, ten years after beginning my medical training, I graduated as a doctor.

JOSEPHINE'S STORY 1954–1983
(BIRTH TO 29)

6

AUTONOMY, INVULNERABILITY, AND A COMMITMENT TO SERVICE

In which Josephine also prepares for her apprenticeship to the culture of medicine, and experiences of trauma, love, authority, power and the nature of knowledge.

Like Patte's parents, my forebears also left their homelands, but several generations ago. They took the risk of months on a sailing ship from Great Britain to a destination of which they knew little. My great great great grandmother was a Quaker and came out to New Zealand in 1837 as a widow, leaving behind her four children, the youngest aged four, in a boarding school. She lived an isolated life in the upper reaches of the Hokianga. Her children all later joined her in New Zealand as adults.

Both my grandmothers went to university in the early twentieth century in New Zealand, which said a lot about them and the men who married them. There was a tradition of service in the Presbyterian ministers in my family tree. My parents were committed to social change and serving the community. Like Patte's mother, mine also trained as a social worker after having a family. She experienced considerable angst about returning to work when my youngest brother was seven, and whether her working full-time was likely to impair our development. My father was a lawyer in a general practice. These days, we do not often think of lawyers as serving us, but he was committed to getting the best for people. I remember him working hard to put his views forward as to how the family court should operate at the time when it was being set up. My parents were both very interested in prison reform. They saw no value in harsh treatment of people who had often had a raw deal for much of their lives. They spoke of the reduction of liberty as the punishment and, in that context, that people should be treated with respect and consideration with a focus on working towards a better future.

I remember my mother talking with excitement about being told, in the context of parenting education, that their role as parents was more like tending a growing plant than moulding clay. Like Patte's mother, she fed her babies on demand – when we seemed hungry rather than to a schedule. This approach

DOI: 10.4324/9781003153788-10

was quite radical at that time. We did have clear boundaries but our parents also listened to us and did their best to support us in making our decisions. They were there for us but there was a clear sense that we could, and would, manage our own lives.

My memory is of a carefree childhood, one of five siblings growing up in a neighbourhood where there were about 20 children living in four adjacent houses, all in their quarter acre (1,000 square metre) sections which were typical for New Zealand suburban life of the time. We came and went freely from each other's houses, returning home for meals when called (loudly) most of the time. Sometimes we would club together and put on performances of singing, or plays and skits we'd made up, for our collected parents to watch. They were an attentive audience. Our summer holidays were at a house by the beach where we swam, played in the sand, took little boats up the creek, and explored rock pools – all with minimal supervision.

The world was perceived as a safer place then but was probably no different from any other time in history. When I was about eight, I was alone on the beach during a family holiday, decorating a sand sculpture with shells, when a man joined me. He offered some shells he had found and we got talking. I felt somewhat special being singled out by an adult like this. He appeared to like me and admire my creation. He put his arm round me, continued chatting and began to touch my genitals. I was a bit unsure but he was gently persistent and I couldn't find a reason to say no. It felt kind of nice in an unfamiliar way.

'You like it, don't you?' he said. Although he was right, I had some sense that I shouldn't like it, without knowing why. We continued to play and talk, with some intermittent touching. To my surprise, he suddenly showed me a long thick tubular thing sticking out of his shorts. I didn't know how to respond. He tried to place my hand on it. I was disturbed and disgusted, pulling back from him. While still having no way to make sense of what was going on, the power of my negative response enabled me to refuse.

'Don't you think you are a bit selfish?' he mocked. 'You liked it when I touched you'.

I couldn't see how to argue with this. As I ran off, feelings of confusion, shame, and guilt arose in me, together with a sense of being vaguely soiled and a bit mean.

These confused feelings surfaced at times in the following weeks. Eventually, I cornered my mother while she was doing the washing and told her about it. She listened but did not pause in her work or make eye contact. She was a bit halting in her responses but said she wished I had told her at the time so that people could have stopped him. This seemed puzzling. How and why they would do this, and what would stopping him look like? Even then I was left with the sense that there was something vaguely amiss with me, rather than that he was at fault and had violated me in a way which had done me harm.

I put the experience out of my mind. When I realised that I should include it in this book, I found writing about it an emotional experience. It was only after a friend who read a draft commented on the disconnected way I had written about it, that I started to process it. Even now, nearly 60 years later, I still have a swirl of disturbing emotions but I can name them now. I know how common it is for children who have been harmed in this way to feel guilt and the sense that there is something wrong with *us*, not with the responsible adult. I can feel for that little girl whose innocent trust was abused by an adult who seemed friendly and kind. I understand how our bodies can respond with pleasurable feelings without our consent. That is a natural, normal process that was exploited by that man. I can feel for my mother who had none of this knowledge then.

I will never know what effect this experience had on my ability to listen to myself and manage my boundaries. I feel sad that I never spoke about it with my mother as an adult in light of what we both subsequently learned in our professional lives about sexual abuse. To have been able to share both of our experiences of this event with the benefit of hindsight could have been the perfect closure.

Right through to young adulthood, I experienced an intense need to protect my parents from being aware of my experiencing any distress or inability to cope. Even now, I can feel a vague anxiety connected with this idea. I remember the horror of the concept of social exclusion being magnified by the thought that my family might *know* if I was socially excluded. Although I cried plenty on my own and with other people, as a teenager I had a longing for my mother to hold me while I cried. This couldn't happen when I was hiding any distress I experienced. My mother died several years ago and I can't talk with her about this but I suspect that she did not need this sort of protection. We had moved past this and I greatly valued her support and companionship throughout my life.

It is common for me with my work now with suicidal adolescents to hear young people describing the feeling that they need to shield their parents, often mothers, from the distress they are experiencing. Their parents' love, and longing to be beside their child in distress, are often clearly visible to me in the room. It fills me with sadness, and I hope that I am able to support some young people to do better than I did. I feel curious about why we try to protect our mothers. As a mother, I do feel my children's pain, but I definitely want to be beside them in it and I think this is a common experience. I wonder how much unnecessary aloneness is experienced, and love wasted, by children and people of all ages, hiding their vulnerability because of a sense that this is necessary for the safety of the people they love.

Growing up in our family, I developed a sense of having a secure place to be myself in the world. In this context I learned to see ourselves and others as having a right to our own ideas and choices. Along with this sense of autonomy was an expectation that I would manage with minimal support. It wasn't that hard. I didn't have to struggle to get what I needed and was very able at school. I was one of those, probably annoying, pupils who could pick

53

up things quickly and achieve pretty well without trying too hard. A number of the teachers in my traditional all-girls school did find my behaviour annoying. I'd not been one to seek trouble. I took a role at home of the 'compliant happy child' but the culture of my family did not prepare me well for the school's hierarchical environment.

School was sometimes mystifying. One Tuesday, a special assembly was called. We were all trooped into the gym. When we were seated the headmistress boomed, 'There is behaviour going on which has to stop!' Not a word more was said, and we all remained in baffled silence for ten minutes before trooping out.

I had several clashes with my teachers which seemed nonsensical at the time. We were required to wear hats and gloves to school. One day I was caught unawares when my Latin teacher held up a school hat, saying, 'Josephine, is this your hat?' Given that we all had identical hats, I asked, 'Has it got my name in it?' The teacher was incensed. 'Don't answer a question with a question!' she replied. Slightly perplexed, I wondered what had upset her.

Another day, the headmistress called me to her office.

'Were you laughing in assembly this morning?' she enquired tersely. I was furiously trying to remember the details of assembly that morning.

'I could have been laughing, but I can't remember', I said in all honesty. At this, the headmistress, like the Latin teacher, was equally incensed and forbad me to go to assembly. This meant I missed something I found rather boring and was able to sleep in, as assembly did not finish till half past nine. The punishment actually was more like a reward. I didn't really consider I had done 'wrong'. I had just been honest and straightforward as my family had taught me.

Near the end of the year, our class was left alone in the music room when the music teacher was delayed until near the end of the period. She was a stickler for punctuality. The words of the hymn we were to sing at prize-giving were written on the board. My friend and I were having fun with our classmates, writing in suggestions they made to change the words. When the teacher arrived she, too, was incensed. As she demanded an apology from me for altering the words of the hymn on the board, I responded by demanding an apology from her for being 32 minutes late for the period. We had a brief yelling match. My 'punishment' was that I was forbidden to go to prize-giving. I couldn't believe my ears as I found prize-giving even more boring than assembly and had been begging my mother to let me stay home. I really enjoyed the TV I watched that night.

My mother wisely shifted me to a more open minded, forward thinking co-ed school where the teachers seemed to find me much less annoying. But in retrospect I realise that these experiences of the foolish use of power in a hierarchical environment were an object lesson of the potential for fallibility of those in positions of authority.

Like my forebears, I have always had a powerful commitment to a life of service. I had planned to be a doctor but I don't remember my family being invested in it. My mother said she remembered my talking about being a psychiatrist when I was a child but I don't remember that. However, at 15, with adolescent omnipotence, I decided that I did *not* want to be a doctor saving people from disease. I wanted to be a social worker, psychologist, or something (it was rather an ill formed idea) and save people from themselves. I gave up chemistry, moved into the French class and left school from year 12 (aged 16) to do a range of arts subjects at university – including sociology, psychology and educational theory.

Going to university in the 70s put me just behind the hippie movement but still into a world where old ideas were questioned. I revelled in the challenge but I don't think the permissive sexual context of the 70s was helpful for me with my limited awareness of my own vulnerability. I engaged in sexual relationships with boyfriends but did not negotiate this particularly well. Writing this, I think of wondering why my mother would want to stop people doing what the man on the beach had done. I did not comprehend the emotional and interpersonal significance of engaging sexually with someone, and the care that was needed. I struggled to identify and advocate for my own needs. I did not understand the potential vulnerability involved in sexual experiences.

My father came into the bedroom where I was in bed with my first serious boyfriend when I was 16. I lay immobile, filled with horror and compassion for my father, wondering what on earth he was going to do. He walked towards us and then left the room without speaking. We had a conversation the next evening – my boyfriend, my parents and I. My boyfriend was professing love and commitment for me. I was out of my depth and wanted out of the relationship but felt unable to speak up for my own needs. I was silently crying. In response to my boyfriend, my mother was repeatedly saying, 'But I don't hear this from Josephine'. This was the end of the relationship and I felt profoundly grateful to my mother for rescuing me by giving voice to my silence.

I started off with my mission to make people's lives better by joining Youthline in 1971. There I was exposed to training derived from the encounter group movement and Carl Rogers' ideas that healing was being present for the person with 'unconditional positive regard'. I enrolled in psychology but the focus in the University of Auckland psychology department at that time was on behavioural conditioning, which did not enthral me. My direction shifted and I became more interested in education and sociology. I loved university. After the limited social world of school with particular groups one could or couldn't be part of, I remember standing in the quad at university and thinking: *I can be friends with anybody here.* Applying myself wholeheartedly to this task, I developed an intense social life and had a great time.

After two years, I felt overwhelmed by it all and decided to go away to a university where I did not know anyone. I was 18. With a conviction that I would manage, I set off to Christchurch with no arrangements for accommodation. Initially I stayed at the flat of an engineering student I met on the plane going down, and found a flat via the student accommodation noticeboard within a few days. For the first time I applied myself to university studies. I bought a portable typewriter for $72 and a spiral bound book to teach myself to touch type. With no social life as yet, I spent evenings working through the keyboard. A good typing speed has been such a great legacy from that time. I wrote essays by literally cutting and pasting. I would write freely, cut up the paper I had typed on, paste bits together and then type out a good copy.

The academic study of education fascinated me with questions like: 'How could you educate without indoctrinating?'; 'What are teachers really doing in classrooms that makes a difference?'; 'How does the human mind develop?' Canterbury had a thriving department with some fine academics. I became swept up in ideas and the pursuit and nature of knowledge. My mother had had an annoying saying that I was clever but not intelligent. I started to understand what she had meant. Suddenly, university was about expanding and developing my thinking, rather than getting the superficial mastery needed to pass exams while spending time socialising.

I fell in love with a young academic who then went away to the University of Illinois to do a PhD. I had been planning anyway to spend a summer in North America, travelling in Greyhound Buses with my female flatmate. We had a great time, met all sorts of people, often travelling in buses overnight to save on accommodation. In fact, when we were in New York City, we took the bus to Boston and back every night and slept in it until we met a policeman in Central Park who invited us to stay in his loft in a warehouse. He vacated his bed for us and slept on the window sill. I did not tell my children about some of these adventures until I felt that they were old enough to be a lot more sensible than I ever was. When we got to Champagne-Urbana where the University of Illinois is, I met up with my academic boyfriend and decided to spend the year there. We had to marry in order for me to have a visa for the year.

Not officially enrolled, I nevertheless joined him in his doctoral programme, engaging actively in many of the classes. Piaget and Wittgenstein were some of our favourite authors. I had already learned about Piaget's work in identifying stages of cognitive development in children. However, I hadn't appreciated how he had carefully watched each of his own children to gain some scientific understanding of how a new baby engages with the world as a model of how humans move towards acquiring knowledge. He observed what a baby's first engagement with the breast can teach us about epistemology.

And as I watch various other species, I still sometimes think of Wittgenstein's question: 'If a lion could speak, could we understand him?' I became almost intoxicated with the challenge of pushing my intellect to its limits with fundamental questions like: 'What is the nature of knowledge?'; 'Is there a world outside our perceptions of it?'; and 'If so, what and how do we engage with it?' An academic career seemed like the only meaningful option.

For the first semester we had both lived, against the rules, in my husband's room in the hall of residence. We spent the summer in Newfoundland where he taught summer school. The second semester we found a job as the 'house parents' of a dormitory in a residential ballet school, developed using sorority and fraternity houses which had fallen into disuse. This was an introduction to grossly disordered eating among adolescents living under extraordinary pressure with very little room for showing vulnerability. Dancing continued despite any injuries. The competition to achieve a paying job in ballet was intense. Being thin was mandatory.

Things were not going so well between my husband and me. This was another relationship I did not know how to leave. I was 21, had no friends of my own in Illinois and no mother there to rescue me. The world was a lot larger then; communication was by letter, and phone calls were rare and expensive. It was hard to know what to say to make the cost worth it. The only phone call I remember was when my parents rang me after receiving a rather flippant letter with a request to be sent marmite, and the information that I was getting married in order to get a visa. Fortunately, although my husband had not wanted me to leave, it was clear that the situation was not working for him either. It felt as if we were making each other unhappy. If I had not had such a clear sense that it was in his interest for me to go, I don't know that I could have. I would have just soldiered on.

I returned to Christchurch to complete my masters, and to do a research project looking at the relationship of the quality of a child's attachment to the quality of their play. I had planned to do observations in the university crèche but, in doing so, started to experience intense anxiety. The staff were very welcoming and supportive but it did not help. I felt out of place there, being neither worker nor parent. I lost confidence in my ability to gather research data effectively, so I abandoned this project without even mentioning my struggles to my supervisor. He was a kind and helpful man with a lot of experience. He might have been able to support me in some valuable life learning if I had been able to share my difficulty. But my childhood knowledge told me that 'not managing' was not an option. If I failed to manage, this must be hidden.

It was June and I had to start again on a research project for my thesis. I had written an essay on the nature of teaching before I went to the US. The essence of it was that *interaction* was central to the activity of teaching – the process of the teacher taking note of the pupil's response and altering their teaching approach. I expanded this into a theoretical thesis. It was the shortest thesis they had ever had in the department but it got a good grade.

Intermittently through these years since I left school, I congratulated myself on not having gone to medical school as the workload of this course would have gobbled up my evenings and weekends. I would not have had time for all the socialising, Youthline, and varied outdoor activities I enjoyed so much. An academic career lost its lustre during the year doing my thesis. I told myself I needed to be in the 'real world'. Without any sense of what direction I wanted to go in, I joined the round of applications for graduate jobs. The job I got was in industrial relations on the waterfront, employed by the Auckland Harbour Board. I enjoyed the colourful characters and the energy in the industrial relations there but administration was not something I could get my head around.

The great love affair of my life began at this time. I moved into a five-person flat. My future husband lived there. In fact, the mutual friend who had invited me to join the flat had felt pretty sure that I would get on with everyone in the flat but felt doubtful about Ian. When I came to meet my potential flatmates, I felt strongly attracted to Ian but thought, oh well, we will be flatmates so that won't happen. However, as so often in my life (and probably everyone's lives), things did not go to plan. I became increasingly drawn to him and within six weeks of my moving in, we were an item. We were immensely happy together, had all sorts of adventures and bought the house we were living in. The months went by in my administration job at the Harbour Board. I still had no idea what my future was. Then, one day as I was sitting in my office in the Ferry Buildings, trying not to while away the time watching the boats, I glanced at the calendar. It was the first of August. 'Damn', I thought. 'I bet the date for application to medical school has passed'.

I hadn't even known I was thinking about it.

7

LOSING SIGHT OF SCIENCE AND WALKING AWAY FROM LOVE

In which Josephine surrenders to the culture of medicine in terms of incorporating institutional knowledge in order to become a doctor and finds herself unable to receive love.

Friends were amazed that I would contemplate another six years of university, but I had loved my experiences of postgraduate academia and was looking forward to it. I was disappointed. In both Illinois and Christchurch, I had been operating in small groups of academics, bouncing ideas off each other, pushing at the frontiers of knowledge and understanding, both for ourselves and humankind. Sitting in a lecture theatre with a class of mostly conscientious school leavers, being lectured on the basics of physics, chemistry, and biology was quite different.

The worst were the labs. We spent hours doing what were called experiments. This comprised following a prescribed set of steps designed to demonstrate something which was already a well-established part of scientific knowledge. This was a parody of science and seemed to me like an exercise in time-wasting. I was not a good lab partner. I got 35% in my first biochemistry test, as I had not realised that what was required was rote learning of equations rather than understanding principles. Not only did I find this uninspiring, but it undermined my respect in the medical school system. It seemed a waste of good minds to occupy them in all this rote learning. These young people did not have any idea of what higher learning could be. We learned nothing about thinking, questioning, and exploring boundaries of knowledge. Hopefully, medical school teaching is more enlightened now, but the reality is that it is a trade training, not an academic exercise in expanding your thinking.

I also struggled with the experience of dissecting cadavers. Occasionally I let myself wonder about the people who had donated their bodies. But at least it seemed an effective way of gaining important learning that would have been hard to do any other way. Despite this, I remained half-hearted about my choice to go to medical school through the pre-clinical years. There was no room for the ambivalence I felt in this exclusive club. I never really

DOI: 10.4324/9781003153788-11

contemplated dropping out but realised how much courage would be needed to leave medical school, once granted entry to the 'club'. I learnt to hide a lot of myself.

In my second year at medical school, I left my relationship with Ian. Like my decision to study medicine, this was another life decision I made in a disconnected way. All I could articulate about the decision was that I felt I needed to leave him to grow up in some way I couldn't make sense of. Our friends were stunned as we were obviously so happy, enjoying our life together.

The years after leaving Ian were a bleak period in my life. I had left the man I loved. He was able to give me a sense of security and nurturing that felt wonderful but uncomfortably unfamiliar. I had broken his heart and, if our friends had to line up with one or other of us, it seemed fair that they lined up with him. As a result, I found myself on the outside of our group of friends. This was exacerbated when the house we had bought, which he still lived in, burnt down. I had loved that house with a passion and had driven the process of buying it. We had scraped together $6,000 for a deposit. The mortgage payments were $30 a week and we were renting out three rooms to flatmates for $11 each. It had been a vibrant five person flat for many years with a strong collective social tradition. We shopped, cooked, and ate communally. Cooking once a week, we each put our all into the meal we made. It was like a dinner party every night. I loved living at the heart of it.

The house burning down felt like a loss to many people who had lived there, had visited and enjoyed dinners. It was a chimney fire. Ian's room was built into the ceiling around the chimney. He woke to smell smoke. If he had been overcome instead of waking, he would have died. Virtually all his personal possessions, including every photo, were burned. He was at the centre of the collective mourning and support around the people who had been living there. Because my presence was painful to him, I completely excluded myself from this process. I felt very alone, with only myself to blame.

8

COMPLETING MEDICAL SCHOOL

Training to Be Superhuman and Joining the Medical Club

In which Josephine embraces the benefits and privileges of the doctor identity, relinquishing awareness of her own vulnerability.

Once we moved into placements in the hospital in the fourth year, my ambivalence towards being in medical school dissolved. It felt as if the entire health system and all the people in it were available to us for our learning. I loved trailing around the hospital in a group of five students in our white coats, following the registrar or consultant who was showing an interest in us. One of my placements was at the cardiothoracic surgical unit, where I was part of the team supporting surgeons sawing through the front of the ribcage with an electric saw, then dividing the tissues to expose the beating heart and lungs.

This was all part of the privilege of being embraced as a budding member of the club. But it was also clear that there was no place for feeling hungry after long hours on the wards, or tired after holding retractors to pull organs such as the liver away from obscuring the surgeon's view. We were in training to be superhuman. I managed as I always had. I learnt to inhabit a sort of artificial self in order to leap into the intimacy of people's lives and the hidden depth of their bodies.

I became totally absorbed in the process of taking histories, with the painstaking detail only a medical student has the time to do. From the perspective from my sheltered life with limited experience of adversity, I felt in awe of how people managed the 'slings and arrows of outrageous fortune' (Shakespeare, 2015). Learning procedures like drawing blood or inserting IV lines on the poor patients, with inevitable failed attempts, was less enjoyable. Being part of a swarm of doctors walking up to a patient's bed, pulling the curtains around as if this provided privacy, and informing them of life-changing issues, gave me flashes of discomfort. I made an error once, during an orthopaedic ward round, by asking a woman how she was. Our job was to review progress with her knee replacement. Afterwards, the orthopaedic surgeon told me that I should never ask a patient how they were – it only invites them to tell you.

DOI: 10.4324/9781003153788-12

61

One of my more sensitive consultants identified the discomfort I experienced in pushing myself into the doctor role. She spoke kindly to me in acknowledging this, but I felt none of her kindness and thoughtfulness. I remember feeling rooted to the spot, paralysed with fear at being found out in inadequacy. My total focus was to extricate myself from the conversation. I feel sad in retrospect for the lost opportunity.

I held a lot of my experience outside of conscious awareness in order to fit myself into the doctor mould that part of me knew I should be resisting. Like Patte, I had also read Ivan Illich and heard him speak when he came to New Zealand. His idea that institutionalised medicine often undermined, rather than supported, health had a ring of truth for me. From my academic studies, I also had an awareness of the potential limitations to medical knowledge. We were learning it as if it were truth, but it was all a construction. It could be argued that it was a construction which met the needs of a powerful and well-rewarded group – doctors. None of this awareness felt helpful. I put aside my capacity to reflect on the process from a more sophisticated framework. I have since learned that the world is full of 'clubs' like the medical fraternity, and many of us give up a lot in order to belong.

Being part of the medical club had many benefits. It gave me an entrée into the worlds of missionaries, aid workers, colonial expats, and local people in Tanzania. We had an opportunity to have three months of our final year gaining medical experience anywhere we chose. I had contact with an obstetrician in East Africa and particularly wanted to get some experience with supporting the birth process, which was difficult to do in Auckland at that time. I arranged to take an extra four months and set off to a small town at the base of Mt Kilimanjaro in Tanzania in September 1983. Coincidentally, this was the town adjacent to the village where Mark's brother had been teaching when Patte visited.

On arrival, I found that the obstetrician I had been corresponding with had left. Knowing I would manage as I always had I was not put off my stride. I took a room in the local YMCA hostel and worked at making contacts in the hospital. Even though I was from the other side of the globe and nobody knew or was expecting me, I was embraced as part of the medical club and welcomed into clinical teams. On the first weekend I took a bus to Mt Kilimanjaro and walked up to the first couple of huts. When I came to return to the hostel on Sunday, the buses were all full. I finally got on a bus but found it stopped at a town close to the Kenyan border and I could not get on another one to complete my journey.

At that time, the border between Kenya and Tanzania was closed. There were acute shortages of many essentials including petrol, cooking oil, soap, and anything else which needed to be imported. Being near to the border the town was generously populated with smugglers and other people living outside the law and, as the light began to fade, I became increasingly uncomfortable. I was aware of a lot of drinking going on in the streets around me.

Fortunately, a couple of young local teachers saw this and took me in to spend the night in the room in which they lived. They gave me their bed and slept on the floor. In the morning, I was easily able to get on another bus. They may well have saved my life. I did invite them to a meal later, but they are some of the many people in my life to whom I have a huge unacknowledged debt.

It was difficult for me to contribute in the hospital. Much as Patte described at the car accident in her blue jumper, I was full of enthusiasm but had little in the way of useful skills. I was further on in my training than she had been at that time, but the skills I did have were in a different cultural context and depended on a level of technical support. Though I knew how to take someone's temperature using a thermometer, I did not have much faith in my ability to assess that by feeling their forehead, particularly in that hot climate.

Every day I looked up at Mt Kilimanjaro hanging in the sky over the town but could not see how I would get a chance to climb to the higher slopes, maybe even the top. I was walking around the hospital campus when a Swedish woman in a Landrover stopped and said, 'Are you Josephine? I am going to Kilimanjaro. Would you like to come? Hop in'. I hopped in. We drove there in about an hour; she did some business and we drove back. This was the journey I had risked my life to make the weekend before.

Thus, began a friendship that greatly enriched my life. She was married to an optometrist on an aid programme to train optometrists and set up clinics throughout Tanzania. They had managed to access petrol and kerosene to take vaccines to a health centre in a Masai area, and kerosene to run a fridge to keep the vaccines cool. Probably the only contribution I made to health in Tanzania was accompanying my friend on this expedition so that a group of children had vaccinations they would not otherwise have had. She would not have gone alone.

We took tents, set up camp and spent three weeks in this remote place as families brought their children in from surrounding villages. Few people spoke English but Swahili was widely used as a trading language, though local people were not fluent in it. I was able to use the small amount I had managed to learn to communicate, after a fashion. We met a young Masai warrior who had not been afraid to engage with a lion, armed only with his spear. But he was definitely afraid of the penicillin injection which would settle the infection in the wounds from the lion's claws in his buttocks.

The local people were as fascinated by us as we were by them. They found our practice of digging a toilet rather puzzling. As nomadic people, they were extremely interested in our tents and would line up to touch my hair, so different from theirs. I may have caused some offence to the parents of a three-year-old girl, who offered me their beautiful little ebony-eyed daughter. I wasn't sure if she was to be on loan or a permanent gift, but either way I had to decline. She looked rather ambivalent about the interaction.

I also accompanied my friend's husband to deliver equipment for the clinics his graduate students were setting up all around Tanzania. Like Patte, I drove round the Serengeti, climbed Mt Kilimanjaro and Mt Kenya, and snorkelled on the coral reef off Mombasa.

The most important lesson for me from this time, in terms of my life journey and the issues we are addressing in this book, was what a lovely person I could be when I was living an engrossing and fascinating life without much stress, and new experiences every day. I was living among people who were missionaries or aid workers who had come to Africa to contribute. Given that, unlike everybody else around me, I felt equipped to make very little contribution to anything, I attempted to be of service in any way I could. In this context, I found it easy to be considerate and generous with my time. The generosity it was so easy to show in this privileged position rebounded endlessly in opportunities. I was invited by a Tanzanian doctor to spend a weekend in his village where I was an honorary man for the weekend. I glimpsed into the lives of a wide range of expatriates, some newly arrived in Africa, some who had full and rich lives there and some who were marooned in a strange country far from home with lives that had fallen apart. This was a magical period in my life. I left with regret, but I also knew that I was only a visitor and needed to return home.

Part 2

BECOMING DOCTORS AND CHOOSING PSYCHIATRY

PATTE'S STORY 1980–1995
(AGES 29–44)

9

THE PLEASANT SMELL OF AFTERSHAVE AND THE IMAGINED RELIEF OF NOT EXISTING

In which Patte finds the resilience to throw herself into the super-human doctor role and love, at emotional cost.

Now that the medical school part of my seemingly never-ending training was complete, it was time to do my house jobs. I began working as a junior doctor in a London hospital. In those days we did 80 hours non-stop on-call at weekends, from Friday morning to Monday evening, plus one in three nights during the week, as well as working every weekday – so having our precious live-in nanny was all the more essential. The focus of the job as a house surgeon was to 'clerk' the new patients. That is, it was my responsibility to take a thorough medical or surgical history and do a top-to-toe physical examination of every patient admitted to the ward while my 'team' was on-call. I was responsible for writing up all the clinical forms, knowing what tests to request, chasing up the blood results and knowing all the various levels of urea and electrolytes, liver function tests, cardiac enzymes, and so on for the consultant ward rounds that occurred most days. Keeping track of those things was my forte. I was obsessive enough to make neat lists and cross everything off as it was completed. As far as I know, I never made an error. No doubt there would have been sleepless nights if one came to light. Thankfully, I was spared this anguish.

In many ways, I really enjoyed being a house surgeon, despite routinely losing a measurable amount of weight each time I was on call due to the stress. I remember several of the people who were under my care in those days. One elderly lady, who knew she was going to die soon, allowed me to put in a chest drain once my registrar had shown me how. She was so grateful for the relief of her breathlessness that she bequeathed me a special treasure from her china collection; a delicate replica of a tiny grey and white field mouse with big round ears. I still have that precious gift along with the memory of how medical procedures can sometimes be so helpful, even if lives cannot always be saved.

In order to streamline my ability to get from my bedroom to the A&E department when I was on call at the hospital, I purchased a pair of black

DOI: 10.4324/9781003153788-15

kung-fu style pyjamas from Marks and Spencer. If I had to get up in the night, which I frequently did, I simply jumped out of bed and put my white coat over the top. No one seemed to notice that I was wearing nothing but my pyjamas underneath. There was one particular casualty doctor, Cameron Doubleton (not his real name) who seemed to be unusually helpful. He was from New Zealand on his 'OE' (overseas experience). He would ring me in the night to let me know that there was a new admission for me. His voice was very gentle and confident, with its lilting Kiwi accent. Usually, apart from saving the patient's life and stabilising him or her, by the time I arrived in A&E, he had already done all the little extra things that the house surgeon was meant to do, such as writing up the notes and suggesting what type of blood samples would need to be taken in the morning. I noticed the pleasant smell of his aftershave lotion.

He seemed far too young to be a doctor but in fact he was less than two years younger than me and a couple of years ahead of me in terms of medical experience, because of the 'detour' in my training. Sometimes he would invite me to share mushrooms on toast that he was making for himself as supper. He would play me his Bob Dylan albums on the old record player in the doctors' quarters as we waited for a patient to arrive back from X-ray or for blood test results to come through. I grew to like him a lot, although we did not have much in common. He was a breath of fresh air around the place. One day at the weekend when we were both on call, he invited me to go for a walk around the hospital grounds. We held hands. He began to ask me a little bit about myself and told me about his recent adventures doing a locum in Thailand, and about his home country. I knew nothing about New Zealand except that it had the Earth's thinnest 'crust' and was prone to earthquakes and volcanic eruptions.

After this unlikely and unpremeditated exchange of intimacy, I did not see him for a while. It was summer. The house-surgeon year was almost over, and it was time I took a holiday. Mark had arranged to have our son for a couple of weeks, and I was wondering what to do. Cam and I had seen each other several times more when on call together over the intervening weeks but neither of us had taken any more steps to deepen the intimacy that had spontaneously erupted between us on our one and only walk together. Nevertheless, I found that he was often in my thoughts. Impulsively, I decided to ring his number and ask if he would like to have a holiday with me; maybe go to Europe together. The phone rang and rang for what seemed like an age. I was just about to give up and almost put the phone down, when I heard a breathless voice at the other end.

'Yes, hello? Cam here'.

'Oh, hello, Cam', I said, rather taken aback at being confronted by my decisive action. 'It's Patte here. This might take you by surprise, but would you like to go on holiday with me? Maybe to France?'

Cam did not hesitate. He caught his breath and laughed. He told me that he had just been setting off to the travel agency to book a ticket to Eastern Europe for a holiday but had left something behind that he needed, so had returned to his flat and heard the phone ringing.

'Yes, Patte, I'd love to go to France with you', he said.

This was the beginning of a wonderful adventure together that was to span the next 25 years. Cam and I set off for France a couple of weeks later in his old orange Citroen with Bruce Springsteen playing loudly on the radio. Over the next days and weeks, as we explored the Loire valley and enjoyed the fresh crisp white wine together in the sunshine, or sat drinking long glasses of cool beer on the Champs-Elysées, we fell deeply in love. On our return to London, he asked me to marry him and I agreed.

I went shopping with my sister at an expensive London department store for my wedding outfit – a beautiful soft-grey winter suit with a wide-brimmed Audrey Hepburn-style hat. I practised having my hair pinned up by my local hairdresser so that it was perfect on the day. I painted my nails bright red to match my lipstick. We were married in early November 1981 in the Hackney registry office. One of my friends, and one of his friends who happened to be touring the UK, were witnesses. We all went to a superb Chinese restaurant for our wedding celebration. My mother was so happy for me. She adored Cam. My son, by now almost seven, accompanied us with a quizzical but accepting expression on his young face. We ate Peking duck, my very first experience of this delicious delicacy.

I wrote in my diary: *Could it be that all my dreams will be fulfilled with this young man?*

It really did feel as if my dreams were being fulfilled. Cam and I both got jobs in a General Practitioner (GP) practice in London and began our GP training together there. I sold my flat and we bought a house across the road in nearby Islington. Cam happily embraced my son while making it clear that he wanted a child of his own as well. Within a few months of our marriage, I was pregnant. Soon after, Cam's mother, who was 53, discovered she had cancer, and he returned to New Zealand to see her for a few weeks. Our baby was born just as I completed my year of general practice training. Cam wanted to take his new family back to his country of origin. We arrived in Auckland in early January 1983. Our intention was to spend a year in New Zealand. The timing of our baby's birth did not allow us to travel sooner, and his mother died shortly before we were able to leave the UK. I felt sad not to meet her.

Cam told me a fascinating little story about how, when he had been in Thailand en route to London before we met, an old Thai clairvoyant had read his fortune when he was visiting an ethnic market. She had told him that he would soon be married and would return to New Zealand within three years with a wife and two children. He had dismissed this as fantasy at the time. And here he was, with a wife and two children.

71

I loved New Zealand from the moment I saw it – the quality of the light, the beauty of the landscape, the dazzling sapphire blue of the sky – so different from the pale blue of London. Even the feeling that we had gone back 50 years in time seemed appealing. Taking time out to be a mother, and to get to know my father-in-law and my husband's sisters, was such a treat. To my surprise, I immediately knew that I did not want to return to England but longed for my friends and family to join us in Aotearoa – the land of the long, white cloud. I wrote endless letters to my mother and my three close friends in London, describing my new life. When our baby son was nine-month-old, it was time for another change. Cam had been doing a GP locum in Auckland. He needed a more permanent position and was keen to support New Zealand's rural community. It was always a challenge to find doctors prepared to work so far away from the main centres.

We ended up getting two three-quarter time jobs at a small rural hospital, one of the most remote in New Zealand, serving an 80% Maori population. In retrospect, I understand what a remarkable privilege this was for a young British woman, to become immersed in a flourishing Maori cultural experience to which few Kiwis ever have access. It taught me so much that I have continued to value. Only recently, since the world events that have overtaken us all with the death in the USA of George Floyd, and the Black Lives Matter movement, have I become increasingly conscious of the complex harmful consequences of the inequity spawned by colonisation. At the time, almost 40 years ago, I was totally naïve about these issues, but I accepted what I saw with an open heart and an open mind.

It took us two days to drive there the first time, with our baby, my older son, and all the necessary equipment, stopping overnight on the way and braving the mostly metal (unsealed) roads for the final leg of the journey. It was culture shock for me and my eight-year-old, moving from London to the tiny community.

In terms of what was required of me as a doctor in my new role, there was so much that I had never done and never seen in my house jobs and my brief GP training in London. There was so much I did not know how to do. The job demanded far more of me than I had been trained to undertake in my two postgraduate years. Really, I was only at the level of a junior registrar, and in England – where the medical hierarchy was much more pronounced – at this stage in my career I would never have been expected to manage so much responsibility. Here, on my days on call, I was triaging, admitting, and treating all medical and surgical emergencies – unless patients were so seriously unwell or injured that they needed to be transferred to the base hospital a hundred kilometres away. Possibly as a result of my own lived experience, I was always very anxious about prescribing medication for fear of causing side effects, so this resulted in many sleepless nights. There was a superintendent overseeing my work, but he was not always on site. Knowing about the management of common problems – such as how to treat a severe nosebleed – soon became essential to my practice. I learned the hard way, calling the ENT specialist at the base hospital for advice the first time I was confronted with my inadequacy. He commented that doctors who did not know how to pack noses should not be working there. I was suitably chastised and embarrassed, but the important thing was that, by following his careful instructions, I stopped the torrent of blood and prevented the poor man from exsanguinating. Thank goodness! I remember thinking at the time that I would look back on all this as a rich and extraordinary experience, but most of the time, with so much responsibility, I found practising medicine as such a junior doctor unbelievably stressful. Fortunately, Cam was always there to back me up if I really needed hands-on medical support.

Part of my job was to help with obstetrics. At medical school, I had done an obstetric run, but only managed to deliver ten babies, which was the minimum required for registration. However, at this little hospital obstetric unit, I always had the skilful oversight and help of highly experienced midwives, who did most of the deliveries themselves. I delivered several babies. As with all the other aspects of this job, it was a wonderful experience, though tempered by anxiety about what could go wrong.

I also gave anaesthetics, assisting the superintendent who performed necessary minor surgical procedures. My 'training' in anaesthetics consisted of three weeks working alongside a consultant anaesthetist at the base hospital in the nearest town, prior to taking up my rural post. As I write this, I feel shocked, although I managed my role without mishap.

One memorably bleak day, when I happened to be the doctor on call at the hospital, and Cam was at home on childcare duties, there was a two-car head-on collision on one of the single-lane bridges. Of the eight people injured, two were babies. One had been thrown against the windscreen and had a depressed skull fracture (a severe head injury). A woman had fractured her arm, her broken bone exposed. The nurses were wonderful and somehow, we managed to address all the medical and orthopaedic needs. This included having to make a rather desperate phone call to Cam, asking him to accompany the severely injured baby in the ambulance down to the base hospital, almost two hours away. Our baby son had to go in the ambulance too.

Somewhere in the mix of memories from that time are images of driving along the winding country roads to attend the outlying clinics and wishing my car would crash. I never talked about that feeling of longing for oblivion with anyone. On reflection, I realise that I never actually admitted these feelings to myself; I did not allow myself to acknowledge the despair and loneliness I felt during this rich and complex time. These unbearable emotions expressed themselves simply in the imagined relief of not existing anymore. Somehow, however, I managed to survive, and in many ways I thrived despite these unbidden shadows.

Cam and I divided our time between childcare, providing medical cover for the hospital, and doing GP clinics in the outlying regions. I was responsible for a small clinic near the coast, where I met a number of wonderful, talented people. Some of them became recognised nationally as major contributors to Maoritanga (Maori culture and heritage). I loved meeting Maori people and beginning to understand aspects of Maori culture. Attending the tangi (Maori funeral) of people whose doctor I had been, was humbling. Because of my doctor role, I had the privilege of sitting with the bereaved family and their deceased loved one. These tangi would go on for three days, and although I was never present for the whole duration, I found the experience totally different from anything I had known. It was very enriching. Occasions of bereavement were celebrated as times of acknowledging and affirming the life of the loved one, with much feasting and singing as well as lamenting, and taking the opportunity and the time to speak about anything and everything that matters. Despite the sadness I felt, I learned a lot from these new cultural experiences.

Overall, notwithstanding the stress and distress, I loved my work and, in particular, the precious relationships I formed with local people. What I found most moving was the trust that people gradually developed in my care as their doctor. Here I was, a young woman from England who knew virtually nothing about Maori culture and heritage, becoming a part of their lives, doing my best to support their well-being and healing. Despite what often began as their scepticism regarding Western medicine, we would engage in dialogue about what was important to them. They would feel heard. One man, a master carver, gave me a beautiful pounamu (greenstone, or jade) carving that he had made. He said it was a symbol of his growing sense of safety, something he had not expected to feel in a Pakeha setting. It is a taonga, a gift that I have treasured ever since, and that I intend to pass on to my sons when the time comes.

Over the two and a half years that I worked there, it gradually became clear to me that my real passion was supporting people psychologically through extreme states. During my medical training, I had done a short stint in psychiatry, but my sense of knowing how to support people through psychosis stemmed from my own lived experience, and from Tony Ryle's human care.

I remember seeing a beautiful, sensitive young Maori woman who had returned home after being hospitalised during an episode of psychosis. As I listened to her story, we made a connection. She told me that the injection she was on took away all her thoughts. She missed the voices that told her what to do; without them, she felt lost. She talked about her isolation and loneliness, and how she had always been bullied by her older stepbrothers, and then by others at school. What she said made sense to me. My impulse was to reduce the 'antipsychotic' medication and see her twice a week so that she could explore what had happened to her. As I listened to her, she seemed to be blossoming. She began to understand herself. The nurse, who was with me in the clinic to administer the intramuscular injection, was alarmed. The young woman had a diagnosis of 'schizophrenia'; she would never recover and needed to stay on her medication, she told me. I was perplexed by the strength of her conviction. She was older and much more experienced than me. In this general practice context, I did not feel confident enough to challenge this perspective, although the dose remained lower and the young woman remained well during my time there. But it got me thinking. Could there be another way?

Cam would really have liked to stay working in this rural setting, and I am sure it would have suited him well. But my older son and I were city slickers from London, and this remote place, albeit so beautiful and delightful in its own way, was not our home. Then one day I happened to read an article in the newspaper about New Zealand's need for psychiatrists. I wondered whether my doctorate in psychology might stand me in good stead to get a position in the psychiatry training scheme in Auckland. I rang to find out. The man on the other end of the phone was Associate Professor Jim Wright. He sounded welcoming and enthusiastic. Before long I found myself making plans, with Cam's support, to move to Auckland to begin the next phase of my life as a psychiatry registrar.

10

WORSE THAN A NUCLEAR WINTER

In which Patte encounters institutional psychiatry with its power dynamics and limitations. The confusing experiences she is facing challenge her ability to make sense of what is happening.

In mid-1985, I began my psychiatry training at Carrington Hospital, an imposing Victorian building that previously had housed a thousand men and women. After my hopes of finding a way to support people with mental health needs, I was horrified that no therapy was available in the acute wards. In my registrar role, I was expected to prescribe powerful tranquillising medication to sedate traumatised people and to sign forms authorising nurses to lock them in seclusion rooms. Our training taught us to talk with people simply to make a diagnosis, not to listen to their stories. Rather than listen to what they were telling us about their lived experiences, we were directed to look for signs in the way that they were speaking that were deemed to indicate that they were 'mentally ill'. I objected repeatedly and loudly to this approach.

Talking with my supervisors about my own lived experience of recovery from psychosis came naturally to me. I felt no stigma. It had been more like some sort of mystical awakening. I felt I had learned a lot and grown in some ways as a result of it. From that time onwards, I had developed what I called 'a sense of pathway'. The extreme state experience had given me a glimpse of an intense reality, one with a dimension including the utter terror of obliteration. But this terror was somehow mystically overcome by total trust and perfect love. It opened a door to a level of meaning in life that was new to me. Discovering the I Ching after this had galvanised my belief in a meaningful reality that was bigger than me. From the age of 24, I took with me a sense that I was going to contribute something that would have that same intense meaning-making effect on other people. I knew that recovery from these states was possible, but not only that; I believed they could bring healing if approached in the right way.

Soon I began to demonstrate a different way of working with people. As in my General Practitioner practice, my model of what a clinical relationship

DOI: 10.4324/9781003153788-16

could be echoed my experience with Tony Ryle. It was what he had inadvertently taught me about the healing power of being humanly present through thick and thin that allowed me to be supportive in this way. Early on in my training I formed strong alliances with two particular women, Clara and Gloria (not their real names), who I continued to see for decades, with the encouragement of several of my clinical supervisors.

I was fascinated by the meaning of the experiences described by the people I met on the acute wards. Often, I found I could help them to piece together what had happened to them, even though I hadn't completely pieced together what had happened to me. I would listen carefully to their stories and I had a natural tendency to validate and normalise their reactions and responses, intuitively helping them to make sense of things. They seemed to rapidly get back on the road to recovery, even when that was not the expected outcome.

Fortunately, in my third registrar job, I had the support of my consultant, Dr Debbie Antcliff, a woman of my own age who agreed that a more psychological approach was preferred. We worked together synergistically on a long-stay rehabilitation ward with adolescents. We were both pregnant with our third babies by this time. It was great fun and exhilarating working alongside her. I was happy to continue with this work for the rest of my life, but of course as a registrar I was required to change to a new position every six months, so it was necessary to move on from there. In any case my baby was soon due.

Then in 1987, almost 12 years after the first extreme state, a second episode occurred. My third son was five months old. I was still breastfeeding and had returned to work part-time. Our house was on the market. My mother was visiting from the UK, staying in a flat down the road. She, Cam, and I had been trying out some philosophy classes. These involved mindful awareness of the here and now, grappling with existential issues of the meaning and purpose of life, and asking the question: Who am I? I was finding this surprisingly unnerving.

Cam and I were in the process of seeking counselling, because we were having some issues in our relationship following the baby's birth. In the midst of all this, the sons of my mother's best friend, whose father had abused me when I was eleven, arrived to visit. My mother was excited to welcome them. I had last seen them as babies and was also happy to see them.

As the date of the counselling appointment approached, I did not sleep well. The day before, a couple had arrived to view the house. One of them was a local psychiatrist I had previously heard was stockpiling long-acting, injectable, 'antipsychotic' medication for his brother, who had a diagnosis of 'schizophrenia', in case there was ever a war or revolution in New Zealand. I was not worried about revolution, but concern about nuclear war was strong in my generation. New Zealand had taken a stand, refusing entry to any nuclear capable warships and this was in the news at the time. I am also wondering now what effect the idea of stockpiling 'antipsychotics' might have had on me, given that they had almost killed me when I was 24.

My mother happened to make a throwaway comment during that afternoon about the philosophy course.

'You'll be teaching *them* when they find out who you are'.

She was probably referring to me having a Doctor of Philosophy degree, but at the time I felt unnerved by her sense of pride in me, and her expectations about what I might achieve.

> *If my mother really knew me, she would die!*
>
> *Momentarily I feel an immense, almost physical weight of responsibility on my shoulders. I see images of being a 'chosen one'. A God; a Buddha; a Christ. A flash of terror leaves me speechless.*

As I cooked dinner that evening, an unusual thought occurred to me. I was making pork sausages and I began to feel uncomfortable about the idea of eating pork. We had eaten pork from time to time as a family, despite the Jewish religious dietary restrictions, but my mother was becoming vegetarian because of her views about the sentience of animals. Her best friend's sons were also Jewish which was raising my consciousness about being Jewish. My two older children were sitting at the table waiting for their food and I began to dish out the meal.

> *I snatch the freshly cooked sausages back off their plates and throw them into the waste disposal unit saying: 'Eating pork is like what Hitler did to the Jews.'*

My older son retreated to his bedroom.

Later in the evening, as usual, I read to the children before bed. We were reading *Mrs Frisby and the rats of NIMH*. In the story we were up to the place where the rats, understanding that they are super-intelligent, realise that in order to escape they must appear to act as if they are merely ordinary rats.

In bed that night I was restless.

> *No sleep. There is a full moon. I am pacing around in the eerie silver light. I am very thirsty. I drink copious amounts of water. I am shivering – my teeth are chattering. I cannot get warm. I am vomiting.*
>
> *This must be the nuclear winter.*
>
> *Terror.*
>
> *My body sensations tell me that this makes sense. Of course. Nuclear winter. I am shocked. I hold my baby boy tightly in my arms. I must keep him alive; I must make sure he does not stop breathing.*
>
> *I must act as if I'm normal.*
>
> *I am in the same predicament as the rats. Fear.*
>
> *That psychiatrist. The psychiatrist who was house-hunting last night, will be back any minute, hunting for me.*

Cam and my mother became extremely worried about my unusual behaviour and called a psychiatrist we both knew. Cam held me while she injected me with haloperidol, a potent 'antipsychotic' medication. Later that day I was admitted to a private hospital in Auckland, where I stayed for two or three days. I was soon back to my normal state and able to return home to my family. I was given a diagnosis of brief psychotic episode and was not required to continue with medication beyond the first couple of weeks. Once again, because of the loving care provided by having support from collegial friends and close family, I escaped the more usual pathway of admission to hospital under the Mental Health Act, and thus, separation from my children.

Although I was able to support the people I served in their recovery from psychosis, my own extreme states took me totally by surprise back then. I had little or no understanding of how they came about or why they happened. It was only years later, during a teaching session when I was using this sequence of events to demonstrate how bodily sensations can be psychotically misinterpreted by the person experiencing them, that a young man who had also experienced psychosis made a comment that brought a much deeper level of insight than I had previously realised.

'Whatever happened to you in real life must have felt even worse than a nuclear winter'.

He was so right! His words helped me begin to make sense of what had seemed a sequence of thoughts, feelings, and actions that could not be understood. The content of the psychosis was not just an arbitrary, meaningless experience. The imagery of a nuclear winter was a metaphor. This was an *aha* moment for me. Following the birth of my third child – because of all the unprocessed events that had come before this – my emotional capacity had been overwhelmed. On some level, my life had felt unbearably painful – as if we were enduring an emotional nuclear winter. The levels of meaning enfolded within the detail of those experiences took many years to unravel and have become increasingly transparent during the writing of this book.

I vaguely knew that what had happened with my mother's best friend's husband, when I was a child, had affected me deeply, but my awareness of the real impact was limited. In retrospect, I wonder if his sons' arrival at the exact time when I was about to engage in marital counselling was just too much for my psyche to process. Rather than facing the impossibility of my predicament, it was more tolerable to dissociate the emotion from the real meaning and to enter into the extreme-state world of metaphorical thinking, and become psychotic.

11

TRUST BETRAYED

Confronting the Devil

In which Patte uses her lived experience of recovery from psychosis to better serve others, with surprising results.

When my third son was around seven months old, I returned to my psychiatry training and continued to work in my rather unorthodox way. There was another brief wobble in my mental health in 1988, following attendance at a personal-growth workshop called *Domain Shift* that was designed to destabilise – and let go of – unhelpful, strongly held, core beliefs. I recall a cathartic outpouring of emotion and rage about what my mother's best friend's husband did to me. Chopping up a vinyl long-playing record of his songs, which he gave to me as a wedding present, released a sense of freedom and relief. Moments after this healing process, the phone rang. It was my youngest brother speaking haltingly from England.

'I have some really sad news, Patte. Our baby has died of cot death', he said. I was utterly devastated.

How can this be? Am I responsible for this horrendous happening?

Immediately I was tipped headlong into reliving the memories of that time back in 1974 when two babies at the crèche had died. I screamed unrestrainedly into the phone, joining my startled brother in his grief. All the loose jigsaw puzzle pieces of trust and fear, death and re-birth, began to resurface once again. I couldn't sleep. I recently remembered a vision from that time:

It is a scene from the future. Devastation. Old and new cars litter the roadside as if cast aside, unable to be used. No air travel is possible. There is danger, a sense of emergency and catastrophe. My oldest son is a man, living overseas and I 'know' I will never see him face to face again except via some form of electronic communication on a screen (this was before the days of the internet and Skype). *He and my brothers are creating a computer program to save the world.*

DOI: 10.4324/9781003153788-17

I voluntarily took some haloperidol after a phone consultation with the private psychiatrist who had treated me after the psychosis the previous year, and who I had continued to see regularly since then. Things settled quickly, and I don't think anyone except Cam noticed that I had been unwell. As always, though, I remained open with my work consultants and senior colleagues about my lived experiences of these extreme states.

Rather than seeing them as something to be ashamed of, I saw that living through them, and trying to process their meaning, was an asset. I believed that it gave me much deeper insight into the phenomena that we were seeing in the people we served. Even though, at this early stage, I had only a limited understanding of the way my early life had impacted me, my lived experience of psychosis and recovery informed my intuition about how to be with the people I served in a more attuned and helpful way.

This was at odds with the increasingly biological understanding of 'schizophrenia' emerging in the eighties. We were being taught about evidence showing brain changes that appeared to correlate with deterioration in function in people given this diagnosis. The apparent effectiveness of what used to be called 'major tranquillizers' and were now known as 'antipsychotic' medication added to the impression of a biological illness. Mistaken interpretation by our senior colleagues of the outcome of psychoanalytic psychotherapy research, carried out at Chestnut Lodge in America (McGlashan, 1984), led to us being taught that such psychotherapeutic approaches were frankly dangerous, and to steer clear of them for fear of exacerbating symptoms. I remember feeling quite concerned not to accidentally cause harm by opening a Pandora's box with the people under my care. However, I found it came naturally for me to form strong connections with each person and listen carefully to their experiences. My lived experience told me that there had to be more we could offer than biological treatments and kindness. All too often, they did not even get kindness within the available services, nor more broadly from 'society' at large.

I had a passion for reading books by people who had engaged in therapeutic relationships with those who experienced psychosis, such as Silvano Arieti (Arieti, 1964) and Frieda Fromm-Reichmann (Fromm-Reichmann, 1950). I made lots of notes from Karl Jaspers' iconic book 'General Psychopathology' (Jaspers, 1964) describing phenomenology, which I devoured from cover to cover. While reading his patients' descriptions of how they felt about their own 'symptoms', I was trying to find echoes of what I had been through. I was finding evidence of hope for recovery and I read much more widely and intensely than was required (or usual) for my training.

One of my sympathetic supervisors told me about a recently published study (Mosher, Menn, & Matthews, 1975; Mosher & Menn, 1978) showing that people with psychosis could do well with minimal medication and the right sort of support. It described a place called Soteria House where people were provided companionship in contrast to clinical relationships and in fact were supported while engaging in normal life activities. In a randomised controlled trial, the Soteria House residents, who were on minimal medication, did better than a matched group who were hospitalised, and often on much higher doses. This evidence of the effectiveness of an approach that stood in stark contrast to mainstream psychiatry was very encouraging as it resonated with my own intuitive way of working.

The Soteria House approach was partly inspired by R. D. Laing who put forward the idea of madness as a sane response to an insane world (Laing, 1967). His ideas had appeared in my life at several different times. I knew nothing about him when I chose his book for my high school graduation prize. I do not remember actually reading it or what impact his ideas may have had on me as a teenager. However, I have a long-standing sense of his having something important to contribute. He happened to be the clinical supervisor of my doctoral supervisor. From him, I learned about Laing's personal limitations and struggles with alcohol but retained my interest in what he had to offer. Prior to the birth of our older son, Cam and I attended a lecture Laing gave about active childbirth. Based on his ideas about the potential damage families could do, he was advocating special care of every aspect of the process of childbirth. Delivery should be as gentle as possible and provide the maximum opportunity for healthy bonding between parents and child. I was impressed by his passion. By the time of the Soteria House research, Laing's ideas had fallen from favour and his work was shunned by mainstream psychiatrists. I found it heartening to see this evidence that he had been right in many ways, despite his personal shortcomings. Some years later, I was compared to him by a psychiatry professor who still held the view that Laing was off track and expressed concern that my ideas were similarly misplaced. But I will come to this in due course.

Despite all the prevailing scepticism of the time, I continued to work psychologically with people in extreme states. *Because* of my own lived experience and the ease and helpfulness with which I intuitively worked with people who were in acute psychotic states, I was formulating psychosis as an understandable response to the person's own unique context. Rather than understanding psychosis as a brain disorder, I was not only conceptualising it as a crisis in meaning-making, of a spiritual or existential nature, associated with great distress, but also with potential to enhance – rather than detract from – personal and spiritual growth. There were times during this period when I seriously considered leaving the training scheme. The approach I was developing was so at odds with the way psychiatry was being practised that I often felt out of place, but my passionate desire to help change psychiatry kept me going.

I was beginning to develop a way of working with the people I served that was clearly helpful in addressing their own self-understanding. I was naturally and gently curious about what had happened to them. Rather than 'assessing their mental state', my intuitive approach was to help them figure out how they had arrived at their conclusions about their world. Usually, they had come into the hospital because there had been some sort of risk either to themselves, or to someone else. Often it would turn out that they had jumped to the wrong conclusions about what was happening, rather as I had. As they pieced it together with my support, they would realise that they could make different, less risky choices, and would soon be on the road to recovery much more quickly than expected. It occurred to me that, in the same way that a muscle could shrink if it was not being used, maybe the brain could literally shrink too because it is not being used. Perhaps this could happen due to the effects of stigma, discrimination, social isolation, lack of occupation, loss of a sense of purpose, despair, hopelessness, and so on. This might explain some of the computerised tomography scan findings. It seemed possible that these changes might be reversible under the right emotional and psychological circumstances. Almost three decades later, the neuroplasticity of the brain was demonstrated on modern scans (Lovden, Wenger, Martensson, Lindenberger, & Backman, 2013). I was ahead of my time.

This was many years before Cognitive Behaviour Therapy for psychosis was developed. It appears that what I was developing has some similarities to this approach. Given that I had a research degree and understood the complexities of the research process from my doctoral studies at Sussex University, I wanted to begin a research project to demonstrate the effectiveness of working in this way.

My current supervisor was Associate Professor Jim Wright. He was the person I had spoken to when I'd made my original phone call from my rural General Practitioner situation, and who had been so enthusiastic about my joining the training scheme. He encouraged me to discuss my approach with him. I had told him about my personal experience of psychosis. We talked about the possibility of setting up a research project. His reaction was that 'this could be the most important breakthrough in psychiatry'. He urged me to write down my perspective on recovery from psychosis. I later did this, handing him an essay titled, *Reframing Psychosis*.

I remember feeling on top of the world in response to his words. That evening I called up one of my close friends in the UK and told her that I felt like Watson and Crick must have felt on the eve of discovering the double helix. The next day I turned on the radio and heard Professor Crick giving an interview about life after the Nobel Prize. This felt intensely meaningful and mysterious – as if there might be something bigger than me that I was part of, rekindling that sense of pathway I had intuited since the episode in 1976. It seemed as if things would fall into place and the purpose of my life would soon be fulfilled. I tried to explain this to Cam. He ended up thinking that I believed I was going to get a Nobel Prize.

Some weeks later, Associate Professor Wright surprised me, almost as an aside, when we were speaking on the phone. 'Did you know that people are worried about your fragility?'

Although I recognised my vulnerability to psychosis, at that time I did not believe it would ever happen again. He went on to suggest that it would be best for me to 'lie low' and complete my registrar training and exams before continuing to develop my ideas or even attempting research. In his view, it would be better for my mental health if I were able to qualify as a psychiatrist first. I found it rather odd that the profession responsible for caring for those who are vulnerable to psychosis should take this attitude to me, but against my better judgement I took his advice, and simply continued with my work as a psychiatry registrar.

A year passed uneventfully. I was receiving good feedback from my senior colleagues about my clinical work. Then my world changed once again. Out of the blue, I received a written summons to meet with Jim Wright and the professor of psychiatry who was currently the director of training. Going on my own, although somewhat cautious about the agenda, I realised we were to be discussing my place in the registrar training scheme.

Shortly after I entered the room, I was told that I was not going to be reappointed as a registrar for the next run. I hadn't seen Jim Wright all year following his enigmatic advice to 'lie low', so I was dumbstruck when he said, 'You're too open, too honest and have too much integrity to be a psychiatrist in Auckland, and Auckland Psychiatry cannot contain you'.

My head began to whirl. He followed this baffling comment by saying, 'It will be a great loss to psychiatry to have you go'.

I could hardly grasp how these sentiments fitted together. The rest of the discussion is a fog to me now. There was talk of research and of my major concerns about the way psychiatry was being practised, which I saw as harmful to people. I made no attempt to hide my disquiet about this. When I got home from this crazy-making interview with the two professors of psychiatry, I looked up the word 'integrity' in the Oxford Dictionary (Fowler & Fowler, 1982), in which it was described as, '1. *Moral uprightness; honesty. 2 wholeness; soundness*'. It seemed to me impossible to have 'too much' of it. I shook my head in disbelief at what had happened. On the one hand, Jim had told me that my theoretical and practical approach could be the most important breakthrough in psychiatry, and that I should qualify as a psychiatrist. On the other hand, I was now being told that I was not to be reappointed as a registrar.

Despite the concerns about my 'fragility' that Jim had mentioned a year before, this issue was not addressed at all in the meeting, nor was there any consideration of my vulnerability in the way the interview was conducted. And following the meeting, I was still expected to be superhuman and do my rostered duty on call that weekend. Thankfully, after a few desperate phone calls, Josephine and other registrar colleagues were able to cover the weekend's call for me. However, despite this support, I was unable to process the enormity of what had happened. Within three days of this interview, having barely slept, I was hurled into an extreme state yet again. The two professors of psychiatry had unwittingly paradoxed me into psychosis.

Hours tick past in a long and sleepless night. I am flying a plane single handed across the world. On board is the whole of the psychiatry fraternity. I am landing safely at Auckland International Airport.

I get up in the morning, I am in a bewildered state. I follow my dog to the nearby park. We are on a time-tunnel trek into my past. The battle between trust and fear rages. I feel a longing for my marriage relationship to be perfect.

Cam noticed me missing and must have called a psychiatry registrar friend to help him once he found me. They took me to the on-call psychiatrist. This happened to be Jim Wright.

Arriving at his office, I kick the door open. I am speaking to him in some sort of foreign language that neither of us recognise.

(Was I speaking in tongues? Or was this 'psychotic' gibberish, speaking out the unspeakable?).

Under threat of the Mental Health Act, I was forced to go to the acute mental health ward in Auckland Hospital, where I had recently worked as a registrar, and where there were patients who I had worked with. Jim later told me that he had tried rather desperately to find an alternative place – to no avail.

I am greeted by two women. They must be my sister and sister-in-law disguised as mental health nurses. (In retrospect I suppose this was my way of managing the terror of being left in the care of strangers). *I lie down flat on the floor expecting that my body will become two-dimensional, and as thin as a layer of molecules so that I might slip out between the microscopic gaps in the walls. The escape attempt fails. I am forced to swallow 25mg of Haloperidol* (an exceptionally large dose by today's standards), *the medication that Jim Wright had prescribed.*

It is night. I am experiencing an intense excruciatingly uncomfortable feeling of internal restlessness. I am being rapidly transported into a place that must be Hell. I am on the brink of being totally obliterated by a massive spherical object the size of the moon, which is approaching me at break-neck speed. Utter terror.

Oh my God - Jim is the devil and he has trapped me in Hell to annihilate me. The black dread-filled sense of obliteration goes on forever and ever and ever.

I did not previously have a belief system that included the devil. Nor did I believe there was a God. But in that lived experience I was confronted by pure evil, with no one and nothing to hold on to; no one and nothing to trust. I was abandoned, surrounded by demonic entities who were hell-bent on destroying me. I have a vague and uncomfortable recollection that, so great was my conviction that I was to be poisoned in this hellish prison, I bit the hand of an innocent and caring nurse as she offered me a paper cup of water along with some medication.

This medication thankfully turned out to be something prescribed by the on-call registrar to calm me down and help me sleep. Mercifully, it worked, and I slept deeply and peacefully for several hours. By morning, the sense of dread and terror began to recede. When Jim came to see me the next day, I had to work extremely hard to figure out that he was not actually the devil. To make sure, I put my arms around his waist and felt the humanness of his body.

'Careful, Patte', he said to me gently. 'You're compromising me'.

Hearing those words, I somehow *forced* myself to recognise that this warm human body must mean that he was simply a man who was doing his best to help me under extraordinarily difficult circumstances. He discharged me from the acute unit later that day or the day after, and I was transferred to the care of my private psychiatrist in a private hospital, where I stayed for several more days. My memory of that time is very patchy, but I know that I continued to take a small amount of medication that helped me to sleep.

The following week I received a letter from the professor who was head of the training committee, explaining why I had not been reappointed.

> The reason for this is not that you are idle, unethical, unintelligent or cannot get on with colleagues or staff. It is that there has been persistent concern amongst your supervisors that your ideas and theoretical models of psychiatry differ significantly from theirs, and from what is considered to be standard practice, in such a way as to raise questions about your ability to practise psychiatry in accordance with what we perceive as New Zealand's needs.
>
> In interview with myself and Jim you intimated that you were prepared to compromise your view of psychiatry sufficient to pass the examinations of the RANZCP, but would not be prepared to keep on doing so in your practice of psychiatry.

The letter went on to state that they had the impression that research was my preferred choice and they wished me all the best in my career outside of psychiatry.

Once again, on the surface I recovered quickly with minimal medication after I left the private hospital, and within two weeks I was back at work. I felt extremely anxious and upset though, about what had happened, and what the future might hold for me now. There would be no further employment offered on the training scheme, but I was expected to complete the job that I was doing. I was terrified that I might lose my hold on reality and was undermined in my role as a psychiatry registrar. My confidence suffered a severe blow. Emotionally I was shattered. How would I regain my sense of place in the world after such an assault on my well-being? This was despite encouragement and positive feedback about my practice, and several letters written spontaneously by my senior colleagues and past supervisors to the Director of Training in support of my case.

I have since discovered that some people on the training committee, including Jim, did not agree with the decision not to reappoint me, but the majority vote won. My current supervisor at the time, Dr Michael Gudex, wrote the following letter to the professor.

Dear Professor......,

Re: SUPERVISION – DR PATTE RANDAL

I am writing both to provide more information than the Registrar Evaluation Form allows, and also to further express my concern over the circumstances around Dr Randal's departure from the training programme in psychiatry.

Dr Randal worked here at .... for 12 months on a part-time basis, the last six months of this time being under my clinical supervision. Both I and other members of the team felt she was an excellent registrar who was able both to fit into and contribute significantly to our team. This was facilitated by her abilities in developing and maintaining good relationships with other team members, as well as her interest in and awareness of psycho-dynamic issues etc. However, her basic medical and psychiatric skills are also excellent, and her diligence and the quality of her record keeping etc have been impressive.

Dr Randal was quite open with me when I first began supervising her regarding her previous episodes of psychosis. She and I were also able to address her tendency at times to take on more of patients' burdens than perhaps was appropriate and sustainable. Nonetheless, this tendency reflected Dr Randal's strong sense of caring and commitment and she had – in the cases where I had concerns of this nature – addressed these to my satisfaction through either terminating cases where appropriate or focusing on specific interventions. I, and other members of the team, found her totally receptive to expression of any such concern, and showing willingness to address such concerns.

I was, therefore, what I can only describe as 'stunned' by the nature and timing of the meeting she had with you and Professor Jim Wright, and by the total lack of formal communication with me as her supervisor, either prior to or subsequent to this meeting. This meeting – and Dr Randal's subsequent decompensation – placed enormous stress on her, but also placed stress on me as her supervisor and on other members of the team, both in their need to support Patte as well as continue working with patients with whom Patte had been working.

I am aware that such courses of action are infrequent and that there is, therefore, perhaps no clearly established process for such action. However, this episode has been sufficiently damaging for all involved that I feel strongly that there needs to be a much clearer protocol which, I believe, should much more actively involve clinical supervisors if their role is really to be seen as in fact of any real importance. I find it difficult to comment more specifically as I still have no clear knowledge of just what event or events precipitated the meeting with Dr Randal. I would emphasise that there was no aspect of her work prior to that meeting which would have indicated such action.

Yours sincerely
Mike
Dr Mike Gudex

In retrospect, I can see that there was confusion about how to deal with my honesty and openness about my experience of psychosis and my perspective about psychiatry. Although I know that the training committee were doing the best they could at the time, it seemed ironic that these 'experts' did not consider that the way they went about trying to protect me, and presumably the 'public' who I might in future otherwise serve, put me at risk. It appeared that I had trusted my previous supervisors too much and they seemingly did not trust me. Not only did they omit to inform my current supervisor about whatever their concerns were, but they also did not stay in a relationship with *me*, or inform me, or ask me, or include *me* in the decision-making. They did not allow me to have a voice. They did not talk *with* me or *listen to* me. They *did things to* me, as if I were fundamentally 'other' than them. I was silenced. I was devastated. It almost destroyed me. Perhaps my spirit was broken. The impact on my marriage was significant. Cam had witnessed my extreme states and experienced first-hand the distress associated with being so closely caught up in them. Sadly, but perhaps not surprisingly, he never fully recovered his trust in my capacity for wellness.

At some point, several years later, Jim made the comment to me that the meeting with him and the professor in 1989 had been 'a stress test'. I can only imagine that he meant this as a cynical retrospective reflection on the way I was treated. I know that he felt really upset about the whole thing and had made an effort to support me.

When I met with the professor in the context of writing this book and asked him about what had happened from his point of view, he said 'I didn't know you. It was a bit like Himmler. I was just following orders'. I took this to be a sort of grim apology from a man caught in a power dynamic that was beyond even his control.

I am aware that we were *all* doing our best in the context we were operating in at the time. Later I adapted the following version of a phrase used in Dialectical Behaviour Therapy (Linehan, 1993):

We're all doing the best we can. And we all need to do better.

The experience of betrayal reinforced my learning about the need for a bridge of communication, inclusion, shared meaning, and mutual trust when working with vulnerable people. I felt a responsibility to speak out for those who had no voice. We all need our voices to be heard. These experiences enabled me, in turn, to continue to apply my personal knowledge with the people I served, with beneficial effect. I began rewriting the essay Jim Wright had encouraged me to write. I called it *Re-framing Psychosis – a New Cartography* and coined the term 'soulosis'. This word portrayed something of my own struggle with trying to make sense of the existential dimensions of the extreme states I had endured. Every time I rewrote this essay, I showed it to Jim, who was very affirming.

Once again, in superhuman form, I did as I was expected to do, and worked until the end of that registrar run. Then I took a little time off work to reflect on my life journey. I decided to try working through my distress by writing the book I had envisioned after my first 'mystical experience'. This turned out to be a semi-autobiographical novel. I managed to find a potential publisher, Wendy Harrex.

'It's a story that needs to be told', she told me.

However, by then I had got it out of my system for the time being and I put it aside. It was that early manuscript that led to the writing of this current book.

Despite having not been reappointed as a registrar, I subsequently got a job as a non-specialist psychiatrist working with 90 people who all had severe and enduring symptoms of 'mental illness'. I was told unofficially that if things went well, I could reapply for a post on the psychiatry training scheme after six months. Initially, I had no intention of reapplying, but then I went to a lecture by Julian Leff who was visiting from the UK. He described his research showing that working with families to teach them how to reduce their critical comments helped to reduce the incidence of psychotic relapse. This rekindled my enthusiasm for the work I believed in. However, my application, after six months of hard and clinically successful work, was turned down. It was clear that the training committee, most of whom did not know me, believed I should not be allowed to become a psychiatrist. No official explanation was given. Despite Jim's earlier question to me about whether I knew that people were worried about my 'fragility', I did not understand at that time that I was being stigmatised and that not reappointing me was discrimination. A couple of weeks after this sequence of events, I was listening to the new album by Tracy Chapman called *Crossroads*. Suddenly, the words from the song *Subcity* hit me like a winter blizzard.

What did I do to deserve this? Worked every day of my life; thought I had some guarantees .... I'd like to please give Mr President my honest regards, for disregarding me, disregarding me.

Those final words reverberated through me, bringing to my consciousness how disregarded, and discarded I felt.

Cam sat quietly with me while I cried my heart out. That was one of the only times in my marriage that I was able to cry. Maybe things would have been quite different if I had learned how to cry more. I bought a copy of *Crossroads* and gave it to Associate Professor Jim Wright.

12

EVOLVING FROM ATHEISM
A Spiritual Emergency

In which Patte reaches another sort of limit and another direction for meaning making emerges with benefit for herself and
others enduring extreme experiences.

Following the second decision not to reappoint me as a registrar, my life suddenly felt derailed, as if the pathway that I had sensed I was following since
1976 had come to an unsurpassable roadblock. Sitting on the steps outside my
house after hearing this news, I felt numb with shock. My two small boys were
asleep in the back of my car. I looked at the pear tree, so recently bedecked
with blossom. An image vividly flashed into my consciousness. There in the
tree, I saw myself hanging, my leather belt around my neck. With that hor-
rific picture in my mind, I turned my eyes automatically towards the blue sky
as a cry came spontaneously from my heart and words formed themselves
out loud:

> God, if you're up there, and I don't for a moment believe you are,
> I need to know right now!!

When Cam came home from work that evening, I told him how lost and
despairing I felt. I didn't mention my unwitting 'prayer'. He then made a proposal that changed my life. Despite his own agnosticism, he suggested I talk
with the husband of one of his receptionists who happened to be the leader
of a small Christian Fellowship. Although I had absolutely no hope of finding
anything meaningful within a Christian framework, I felt I had nothing to lose.

Agreeing to meet in his office, this friendly man asked me some questions
about my spiritual life. I told him how I had relied on the I Ching to help me
find my sense of pathway. Recently I had stopped using it after coming across
an article which revealed that for all those years, ironically, I had been using
the coin-throwing formula wrongly! It made me laugh. I had been doing it
back to front all that time. Nevertheless, the readings had always brought such
a sense of meaning for me. After I told him about these activities, he opened

DOI: 10.4324/9781003153788-18

a big black Bible that was on his desk, and quoted me a scripture from Isaiah 30:15, emphasising the second sentence:

> In quietness and confidence is your strength. *But you would have none of it.*

I'm sure he was trying to encourage me to change my ways. Ordinarily I would have rejected any suggestion that I might read the Bible, but these were not ordinary times. After this, he suggested that I throw away the I Ching and read the Gospel of John. Given my doubts about the I Ching, I agreed to do this. Then he prayed a simple prayer for peace. I left feeling calmer than I had for days.

Several days later I visited Gloria, one of the two women who I had continued to see in my doctor role through all the ups and downs over the years. She happened to be back in Carrington Hospital. Dressed in a green towelling bathrobe, her long brown hair falling over her childlike tawny eyes, she was rocking back and forth, distraught. As I placed my hand on her arm, her demeanour changed. Relief. For some strange reason I offered to pray for her. I guess it was in the spirit of medical-school training where the edict is 'See one; do one; teach one'. I prayed the same prayer that had been prayed for me, the unfamiliar words coming to me slowly as I tried to recall the gist of what he had said.

> May you have a sense of peace and may you be comforted in a way that goes beyond your own understanding.

'Thank you', said Gloria haltingly. After a few moments she settled into her chair, a bemused grin beginning to light up her pretty face. 'I feel much better now'. She went on to tell me that the doctor in the hospital had asked her that day whether she had a personal faith and had suggested she receive pastoral care when she had answered in the affirmative. Later, returning to my car to drive home, I turned on the National Radio programme that I always listened to. Words from a popular song by Alison Moyet that I had never heard before hit my ears:

We all need a little Divine intervention.

I gasped, feeling breathless. Those uncanny words made me smile in amazement, a bit like Gloria had just before. I thought of my heartfelt out-pouring of desperation only a few days previously, asking for evidence of 'God' – something or someone bigger than me that might somehow help me. Was the God – who I believed did not exist – responding to my heart cry? As it dawned on me, the possibility felt tantalising.

I had been grappling since the years of my doctorate with the concept of 'truth'. I had tried to figure out the place of the scientific method in discerning what is 'true'; explored acupuncture and Taoism; used the I Ching divination process to 'magically' and irrationally help me find a sense of direction. I had found myself in mystical places where cosmic truths about trust and fear seemed self-evident, and yet then had to discover all over again that gravity still exists even when my inner world was turned upside down.

As I began reading the Gospel of John, the veracity of the story about the young Jewish man, referred to as Jesus, somehow reached me. It was as if the author was telling it as he experienced and believed it. His truth. It occurred to me that the Bible was still used in law courts when people chose to 'swear to tell the truth, the whole truth and nothing but the truth'. Could the story told in *this* ancient book somehow represent 'truth' in some way that I was yet to fathom? But this was no sudden Damascus Road conversion experience for me.

In the weeks that followed I began to attend the little Christian Fellowship that met in a local school hall. Every time I walked in, I found myself weeping. Something about the experience of being among these people, their prepared-ness to be open and believe, was humbling. I felt a sense of trust. I decided to read the whole Bible, every page, Genesis to Revelation, eventually getting through it five times from beginning to end. I found it fascinating. The Old Testament contained the Torah that my mother had told us about, with all its shocking stories of life in the raw. Incest, rape, adultery. It was all in there. Because she had been so scornful about the mistakes in translation, I did not spend much time on the King James Version. I read more recent editions with historical notes, and books with titles like *Reading the Bible for all it's Worth*. Initially, it was an intellectual activity – getting to grips with my spiritual heri-tage. A lot of it seemed to be a metaphor, interspersed with interesting facts. A novel called *The Light that was Dark* seemed particularly illuminating, regarding my foray into New Age thinking, with my erstwhile obsession with the I Ching.

Despite my unbidden brushes with a mystical dimension, it took me many, many years of study and reflection for my basically atheist, secular, humanist worldview to begin to evolve, and for my mind and heart to become open to a more spiritual perspective. In the past, the scientist in me always wanted to have the final say. But over the ensuing years, the words of scripture began to speak to me. From my point of view, given my Jewish roots, I was becoming a Jewish follower of Jesus (or 'Yeshua', his Jewish name). But I think my mother felt she had lost me. She just wanted to dismiss it. I recall her saying to me: 'It's a pity you found Christianity before you found Judaism'.

Prior to this, she had adulated me and my choices. Our approach to life had somehow been merged. She'd always wanted me to follow whatever path I chose, but she never wanted to know about this part of my life. It was shocking to her, as if I had joined a cult where you allow your own thinking processes to be subsumed.

She had seen her mother's limp body thrown into the grave when she was nine. It was horrifying. At that point she gave up on engaging in the religion of Judaism. As an adolescent she was a communist, then a socialist. Lately, while in New Zealand, she had been exploring her identity and joined a Jewish women's group, becoming friends with strong, contributing women such as Marti Friedlander. She wanted me to embrace something similar. But it was time for me to find my own way, separate from hers.

All through this time, I continued to support Gloria and Clara, both of whom had chosen to engage with me in my therapeutic 'being with' role as a registrar, and subsequently as a non-specialist psychiatrist. Neither of these women was any better for all the frightening diagnoses, toxic medications, and stigmatising experiences they had endured within 'the system'. Both had histories of unbearable trauma in their early lives and it was clear that each of them benefitted from the therapeutic connection with me. I couldn't just abandon them as I had been abandoned by the training committee.

A special source of funding became available to enable me to continue supporting them. Tony Ryle's way of being with me gave me permission to be flexible in the way I offered a therapeutic partnership. I always had consultant psychiatrist oversight in this work, and my approach was valued and clearly effective. Albeit a very unusual step, in consultation with my supervisor, I invited them to come along to church with me, an offer which they both enthusiastically took up. My focus in their company was always on their need for companionship and social safety, rather than on reciprocal friendship. By now, I was neither their psychiatrist nor their therapist. My role took on more of a mentoring style. We all enjoyed immensely our new-found community and fellowship – the singing; the teaching; the prayers; the cakes and coffee afterwards. We were embraced wholeheartedly by the others in the church, with no questions asked.

Eventually, Gloria and Clara became firm friends and supported one another as peers through many subsequent years. They often told me how much they enjoyed spending time together. Both were exceptionally talented in many ways, including being artistic and creative. It became noticeably clear that their lives were enriched by their mutual care and the fun they had with each other. Sadly, Gloria died of cancer almost a decade later. It makes me happy to know that the last years of her life had been enhanced by this special friendship. Clara still contacts me from time to time to let me know how things are going for her. It's been over 30 years since we first met. I value her as a person of great warmth, courage and endurance, and I always enjoy seeing her when she gets in touch. Over the years that followed, I developed a number of peer mentoring relationships with people who were referred to me by psychiatrists. Several of these were doctors who, like me, had experienced extreme states.

Back in those first weeks at the little Christian Fellowship, we were learning new songs from an album called *Combat*, all about 'spiritual warfare'. The words of one particular song spoke to me, from Ephesians 6:10–12.

'Be strong; put on God's armour, cos we're not fighting human enemies, we're fighting a war in the spirit'.

These words resonated with me because of my long-held sense of a hidden cosmic battle. There had been occasions in the midst of my extreme states when I sensed a massively overwhelming force was hell-bent on obliterating me. This was certainly no human enemy, but it felt like the enemy of my soul. After the service, I read the scriptures mentioned in the song and noticed that in Ephesians 6:11 it says:

> Put on the full armour of God so that you can take your stand against the devil's schemes.

I had briefly held the belief that Jim Wright was the devil, although soon realised he was neither Satan personified, nor my enemy, but a human person doing his best in dire circumstances. Even though I did not even believe in the devil, it's as if I had confronted a devil-like cosmic destructiveness before I had any solid sense that there was a transcendent, loving, trustworthy context bigger than us. I had experienced time stopping and an eternal now that on the one hand was utterly terrifying, and yet, somewhere in my psyche or soul, there was also a 'knowing' that ultimately, trust overcomes fear.

The following Tuesday night our church group read the same Bible passage in Ephesians and we discussed what all the parts of the armour meant. Before falling asleep, a paragraph jumped out at me from the book I happened to be reading (by a Swiss doctor, Paul Tournier), which referred to our need for protective spiritual 'armour'. The next day, I was in my car driving along Balmoral Rd in Auckland, praying and thinking about this scripture and all the parts of the armour, and why this felt so relevant for me in my current circumstances. I had stopped at the traffic lights when a man appeared, as if out of nowhere, and asked through the window, 'Do you read the Bible?'

Looking at him in stunned silence for a second, I blurted, 'Well I've been reading it for the past few weeks. Why?'

He handed me a small white piece of paper on which were printed, in bold black letters, a list of the exact same phrases that I had been reading and singing about:

The Full Armour of God;
helmet of salvation
breastplate of righteousness
belt of truth
shoes of peace
shield of faith

sword of the spirit (the word of God)
Prayer
Do not leave home without it.

(See photo of this piece of paper on
www.talkthatheals.org)

Taking the paper from him, I felt so stunned that I had to park my car and take a few deep breaths. Later I would joke, 'Could it be that not only does God really exist after all, but S/he sent me a letter!?'

Receiving that simple piece of paper was like the in-my-hand manifestation of the existence of God. The way the coincidental sequence of events unfolded made it feel as if the 'little Divine Intervention' that the song said we all need was happening live in my here-and-now world. The revelation that being in a 'spiritual battle' was a biblical concept gave me a way of understanding what was happening to me. It was a new concept to me that I might have 'an enemy' in some spiritual sense. Since childhood, I had been harmed by trusting everyone implicitly, and not knowing how to protect myself from untrustworthy relationships. But, as it says in the song, I was not fighting human enemies. I always had compassion for the people who had harmed me, trying to see things from their perspective as well as from my own. As I learned to meditate on each of the parts of the 'Full Armour of God', it was to take on profound meaning for me, making a tangible difference to my life over the coming years.

The metaphor taught me how to protect myself on many levels. I learned to be more mindful of my bodily responses alerting me to stressful situations. I began to be more resilient, always asking for divine help and guidance when I needed it and being thankful when I received it. Eventually, when I later learned the mindfulness body scan in my professional role, I realised that it lends itself to a 're-minding' of the 'Full Armour of God', with its emphasis on bodily awareness from head to toe (helmet to shoes). After this, I became much better at 'putting on the armour' of peaceful awareness in the midst of upsetting thoughts, and the uncomfortable body sensations in my chest which denote anxiety. Hopefully this helps me make wiser choices. The first scripture that had been mentioned to me was becoming a reality.

'In quietness and confidence is your strength'.

Around this time, I was invited to join Life Unlimited, a Christian Counselling organisation. As part of my orientation to my new job, Charlotte and Liz, who set it up, encouraged me to participate in a course they ran called *The Divine Plumbline*, where I learned another pivotal biblical concept. The idea was that any behaviour or thinking that is out of alignment with the 'plumbline' of Jesus' teachings about love would inevitably result in negative psychological consequences. Mental health and well-being could be found in alignment with loving relational experiences including unconditional love, acceptance, affection, discipline, and guidance, along with developing capacities such as self-control, love, gentleness, joy, and peace.

Recently I found the workbook that we used during the course, a large yellow children's scrapbook filled with my drawing, diagrams, personal reflections, and brainstorms. It's fascinating to see what I learned during that enriching few weeks back in 1992–1993. Each page detailed the goals of the course and my subsequent reflections on these. Looking at the notes I made reminds me that this group context allowed me to identify, in a safe environment, some of the traumas I had endured. It provided a meaningful framework for processing and finding growth in these experiences and was to form the groundwork for my future clinical work.

The notion of the Divine Plumbline included figuring out what factors had created 'the walls of my heart' (or, my defences). This helped me identify the unhelpful ways of coping I had developed, such as suppressing feelings, withdrawing and meeting others' needs rather than my own. I learned about the power of prayer, particularly writing out my need for help, and receiving hope-inspiring messages from others, or from certain scriptures. However, I also found that prayer was scary in some ways. How would I deal with the disappointment if my prayers weren't answered? Would I lose my budding faith?

What stood out for me, though, was the way that, time and time again, despite the reality that almost always things were not as I hoped, my sense of well-being deepened as I felt held by a mysterious, loving force. My time working with this supportive organisation was filled with moments of joy and gratitude. From then on, I incorporated this basic framework into my therapeutic stance, and looking back I can see that it became the foundation upon which my future rested.

During the plumbline course, we were encouraged to draw a timeline of significant life events, going from birth to the present. As I reflected on my life, with all its ups and downs, it appeared to have no particular pattern or meaning. For me it seemed just a random sequence of events, that would go on until death, getting nowhere. Suddenly I recalled that a couple of years earlier, a psychologist friend who was trying to help me understand what had led up to my second and third episodes of psychosis, offered me an *aha* moment.

'Life might not be a linear process', she said. 'It might be a spiral'.

It made sense. There definitely was an impression of things repeating themselves in a rather uncanny and meaningful way. Somehow this image added to the sense of pathway that had felt so hope-inspiring. It felt as if I found myself on a cosmic spiral staircase, bringing meaning and purpose to what had happened to me, onward and upward.

Example of a spiral I drew in 1990–1991 (see Figure 12.1).

In therapy sessions with people, I drew rough diagrams of this spiral process, looking at ways we could support a more successful negotiation of the patterns that kept re-emerging. Eventually, I coined the word 're-covery', with the hyphen between 're' and 'covery', to describe this process of covering and

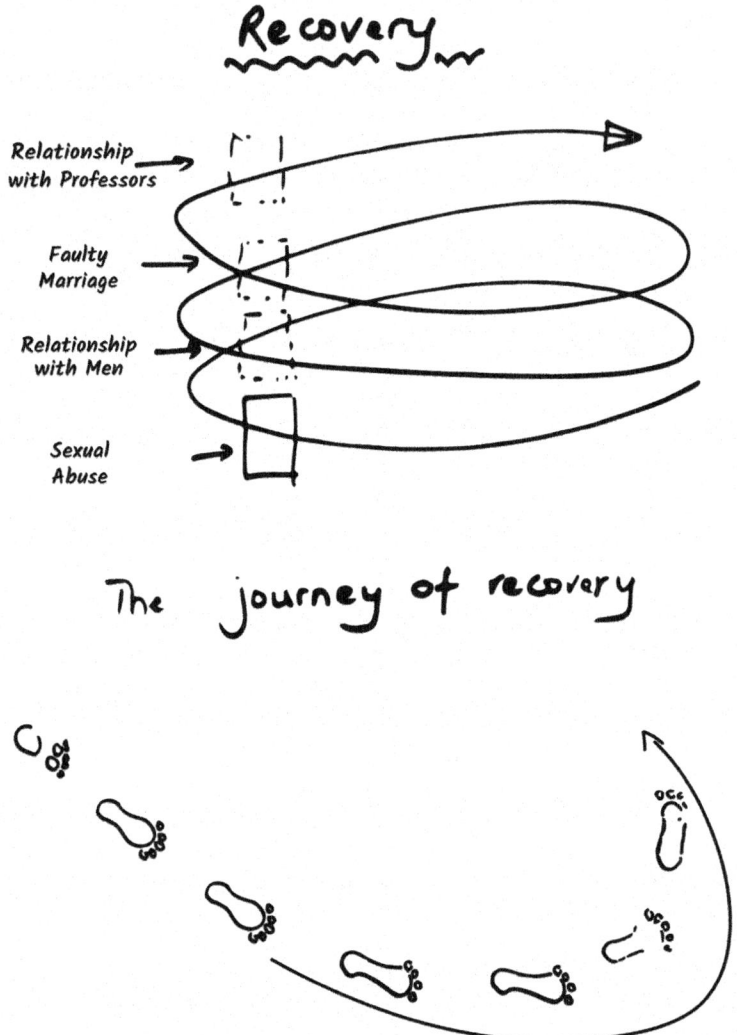

Figure 12.1 Example of a spiral I drew in 1990–1991.

re-covering the same old ground. I would often reflect with people on the ways that, metaphorically, it might be possible to 'put on the Full Armour of God' in order to have protection from the vicious cycles that might otherwise be perpetuated. Our spiral life journeys give us the opportunity to 're-cover' old ground in new ways, always learning as we develop more effective ways of coping. This was the beginning of what eventually became *The Re-covery Model* that was published in 2009 (Randal et al., 2009).

I was loving working at Life Unlimited, preferring to be under God's authority rather than the authority of psychiatry. However, in 1993 through a contact in the Christian Fellowship, I met an academic lawyer and told him my story. He said that I had a legal right to contest the decision that had been made not to reappoint me as a psychiatry registrar. As I thought and prayed about the implications of this, I had a change of heart. Maybe my pathway was to become a psychiatrist after all. I wrote a letter to the then chairperson of the training committee, explaining my position and letting him know that I had the support of the associate professor of law in asking to resume my training in psychiatry.

To my great shock and surprise, I soon received a response to my letter, telling me that I had been accepted back into the training scheme. It was as if nothing had happened. There were no questions, no concern expressed about my vulnerability to becoming 'psychotic', or about my ideas or theoretical frameworks. There was simply an acknowledgement of my letter and a proposed starting date. The rug that had been inexplicably pulled out from beneath me was equally inexplicably shoved back in place. If being thrown out of psychiatry had made no sense, this reversal made even less in my naïve and trusting mind. It was as if the pillars of society suddenly turned to dust and collapsed. My reaction was to stop sleeping and, within a short time, I was once again re-covering old ground in yet another tipped-up jig-saw puzzle episode, unable to piece together the meaning of this bizarre sequence of events. For the fifth time, I found myself in the grip of an extreme state.

Night.

I am terrified that there will never be another sunrise. The sense of relief when morning comes is beyond description. There is a big party taking place at the medical school and my work is being celebrated. I am dying. I am being re-born.

I am sitting around the table with Cam and my friends, Liz and Charlotte, eating a meal together. The food is made of solid gold and we are mystical kings and queens.

I am making colourful drawings in my notebook, writing out scriptural messages that have special meaning for me (see www.talkthatheals. org). *It is around the time of my birthday and I write:*

'Happy Birthday Death Day.'

I am drawing a picture of Jesus on the cross and another of a three-dimensional hysteresis loop, surrounded by the words:

'Darwin's theory of evolution. Survival of the most loving. Parallel evolution of species with each new generation (evolution of consciousness; physical evolution is now completed). We are the chosen generation. Look at the structure of the brain; lateral ventricles, third and

fourth ventricles. The brain is a flexible, living organ, responsive to many internal and external influences. An oscillating system of fluid dynamics.'

On this strange three-dimensional picture, I depict the pendulum swing from misinterpretations of pleasure, pride, mania, grandiosity on one side to pain, unbelief, rejection, paranoia, and depression on the other side, with the divine plumbline as the place of alignment in between, representing love, peace, joy, gratitude, kindness and patience. I write:

'God's plumbline: Jesus/Yeshua the man'.

'Re-covery Process; rebalancing neurotransmitters. We need to align ourselves with one another in love. High expressed emotion = feedback that pushes the system out of alignment'.

'I am a wounded healer. This means I may wound others. Father protect them and me'.

I am drawing lots of coloured pictures of myself and others with little flames representing the Holy Spirit somehow linked to the ventricles. I draw upright flames aligned with the 'divine plumbline' of self-control, gentleness, love, joy, and peace.

I write:

'I am essentially a sinful person capable of horrible thoughts and feelings. I am not perfect. Father forgive me for believing I was someone special in my own right. Cleanse me please and allow me to be holy; a priest for You'.

I am drawing a picture of a swirling black vortex surrounded by frightening ghostly figures labelled 'death', 'deception', demons', 'fear', 'delusion', 'depression', 'mania'.

I write:

'Who, what, is Satan? He was a murderer from the beginning, not holding to the Truth, for there is no Truth in him. When he lies, he speaks his native language, for he is a liar and the father of lies. He robs. He destroys. (See Figure 12.2 showing a picture I drew depicting 'Who, what is Satan?').

On another page I write:
'Your crown of thorns will become a crown of jewels.'
I am drawing a picture of myself wearing a purple gown, with a crown on my head.

Poor Cam was upset by my odd behaviour, called my private psychiatrist and accompanied me to see her. She prescribed small doses of an 'antipsychotic', which dropped my blood pressure, making me very dizzy but helping me to get some much-needed sleep. Some lovely people in the fellowship group invited me to stay with them in their charmingly rustic home in the countryside for a few days respite, so that I didn't need to be hospitalised. They shared helpful,

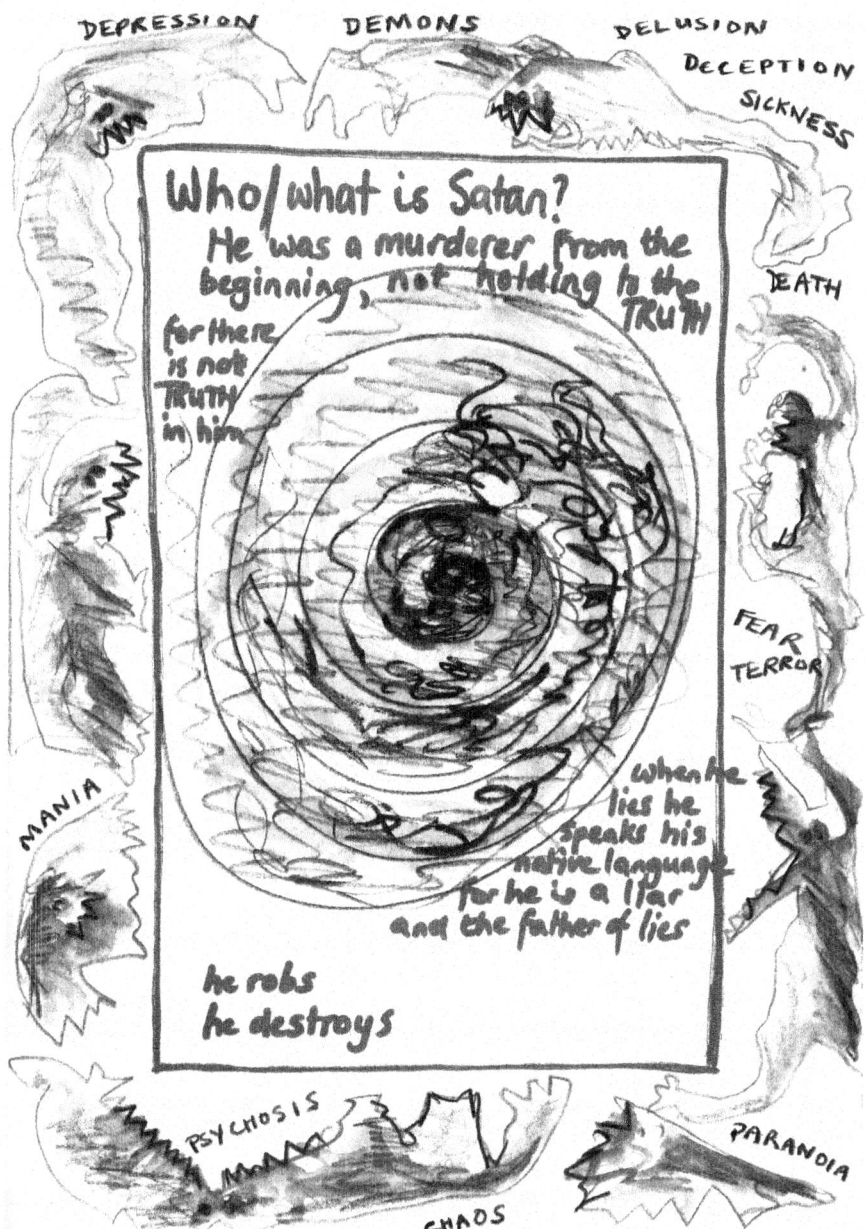

Figure 12.2 Who, What is Satan?

hope-filled scriptures and we prayed, sang, and ate together. They were able to be with me in a way that was nourishing for my body and soul. It made me feel secure and safe. Although there was joy for me and my new-found friends, this crisis – which had become an opportunity for spiritual growth for me – was undoubtedly a very frightening experience for Cam and my boys. Better for us all that I could be away from home during this time.

There was something redemptive for me about this whole episode. A scripture stating that 'God did not give us a spirit of fear, but of power and love and a sound mind' felt strengthening and grounding. I began to realise that the context in which we live and move and have our being is indeed loving, rather than the terror-filled darkness of the extreme states. Soon I was able to return home and took whatever steps I needed to at work, to prepare myself and the people I was seeing, for my departure from Life Unlimited. However, I felt perplexed about why this episode had happened. Now that I was developing this new faith perspective, I wondered why a loving God would allow this to happen again. Was I doing something wrong? Could my faith protect me from another episode?

Looking at the pictures and writing in my notebook, a friend remarked, 'Sometimes God lets the devil overplay his hand'.

Although I did not take it literally, this idea was surprisingly helpful. It linked back to the spiritual battle against 'the devil's schemes' that I had read about in Ephesians 6. I could see that what had happened could make me think that I was lost; that repeated episodes of psychosis, fear and doubt were to be my lot in life. But now the 'devil's scheme' was being revealed to me so that I could resist this untrue belief that had been sown in my mind, and find a life free of psychosis, fear and doubt. God had not given me a spirit of fear, but of love and power and a sound mind. While staying with my friends, I had learned scriptures that said, 'Resist the devil, and he will flee from you', and 'You belong to God and the battle with the enemy is already won'. These illuminated even more clearly that I needed to mindfully 'be still' and 'draw close to God', by seeking shelter and protection in spiritual practices such as prayer; finding meaningful stories, words, and phrases that I could relate to in scripture readings; and attending the Christian Fellowship. Hopefully, this would help protect me from another extreme state episode.

From that time on I have built these disciplines into my daily rhythms. I began to keep a prayer journal. Whenever times of anxiety or fear arose, I would have a written conversation with 'God' about it. It's not that I literally thought any outside 'person' was interacting with me, but there is a mystery to it all that somehow feels comforting, as if I am held by an invisible presence. After my first extreme state, I had found it helpful to reflect on what had happened by journaling. Now, writing as prayer became my way of seeking comfort and meaning within a bigger picture, in which we are all composed of star dust and are evolving to love one another as we are loved. Although my spiritual approach has become more contemplative over time, some of these original practices continue to this day. For example, if ever I have difficulty sleeping, I write down what I feel grateful for, and detail all my concerns, worries and reflections, prefacing them with the words, 'Loving God, as You know …'. Then I write, 'Thank You that You give Your beloved sleep', and almost always fall into a peaceful sleep.

Josephine tells me that nowadays not only is gratitude journaling at the forefront of positive psychological intervention research, but it has also been found to be associated with brain changes (Karns, Moore, & Mayr, 2017). It's exciting to realise that there is hard evidence for the effectiveness of a strategy I have personally found so helpful. But for me the spiritual component is even more important. I recall the utterly surprising thrill and awe of experiencing what felt like evidence of 'God' showing up when I least expected or believed in that possibility. I do not believe I would have been able to manage my life and thrive without having believed that as my reality at that time. In turn, this perspective has taken a role in how I have continued to serve others in my work.

Before I returned to my registrar position, I was open as always with the training committee and my prospective employers about what had occurred. It was becoming clearer to me that these episodes could happen under certain circumstances, although I didn't understand the detail of how this came about. To my amazement there was no vocational fallout this time, despite the now overt reality of my vulnerability and the way it could potentially affect my ability to practise my profession. I simply was required to develop a plan of action with my psychiatrist to cover the options of what I would do if similar circumstances were to recur (a kind of advance directive), which seemed a very good idea to me. I was given the go-ahead to proceed with my training to become a psychiatrist.

It never occurred to me until we were writing this book that the training committee might have been concerned about legal reprisals. I always find it hard not to trust people even when they have shown that they are not trustworthy. It is part of my nature to see the best in people, and not to be cynical. Friends suggested that the committee let me return to the training just because I had the support of a lawyer. I still find that hard to believe and if it is true, I feel disappointed and sad about it, even though the outcome has been beneficial.

13

DEFINING THE ESSENCE
OF PSYCHIATRY

In which Patte experiences more challenges, success, failure, support, overwhelm and hope.

So, the pillars of society had crumbled and here I was back in this system where nothing stood up to scrutiny. My intention was to complete what was left of my training in as short a time as possible. It was no joke to be in the Auckland psychiatry training scheme once again after a three-year break, especially as my first placement was in child psychiatry under the professor who had headed the training committee that had thrown me out. I feel sure that it was no coincidence that he took on the role as my supervisor. I didn't feel that he had anything personal against me, but I wondered if I had been 'placed' in his unit in order that he could observe and direct my practice. He welcomed me back with seeming warmth. When I arrived, I talked with him about the episodes of psychosis I had endured, as specified in my voluntary undertaking.

'Have you had a falloff in function?' he asked.

Was he questioning me to establish whether these psychotic episodes represented what he might diagnose as 'schizophrenia', or some 'milder' form of 'mental illness'? A deterioration of function is a requirement for the Diagnostic and Statistical Manual of Mental Disorders diagnosis of 'schizophrenia'. Looking back, I can see this was inappropriate in the context of the power dynamics in the role relationship. At the time I found it both interesting and frightening. I checked back over my memories trying to fathom whether indeed there might have been a 'falloff in function'. I seemed to be managing the juggling act of my work plus my multiple roles as a wife, mother, and friend in much the same ways as I always had, despite times of extreme distress. But how could I be sure?

After each episode, I had quickly recovered enough to look as if I was back to my usual self, but there was always an enormous process of repair needed on the inside. It was a struggle to get back on my feet. Initially, when I woke up in the morning, it felt like an achievement to open the curtains.

104   DOI: 10.4324/9781003153788-19

I wasn't sure that I would be able to do much else. Standing outside the school gate, waiting to pick up my children, I dreaded the possibility of somebody speaking to me. I was able to appear to function on the outside. But underneath, after each episode, I had lost my confidence in the world. It was almost as if I had lost my elastic.

When I thought about the question the professor asked me, sliding down the slippery slope towards losing the ability to function seemed so easy. There but for the grace of God go I! I have often wondered what might have happened to me if Tony Ryle had not been so courageous in his management of my care back in 1976. If I had been 'sectioned' under the Mental Health Act, medicated and relegated to a ward in the local asylum at the age of 24, I may well have lost all hope, given up on life and developed what might look like the so-called negative symptoms of schizophrenia. Could I have ended up in a back ward, or eking out a lonely existence in a Sussex boarding house? Could I have killed myself?

Notwithstanding this rather unnerving start, the professor and I seemed to get on well professionally, albeit in a slightly awkward way. It was all very odd. I managed to fit myself into the routine of the ward and did my work as well as I could for the required six months. I even managed somewhere along the way to win the registrar Grand Round Prize for a presentation about someone I'd seen on call with a curious and rare condition characterised by hoarding rubbish, severe self-neglect, social alienation, and refusal of help. I felt compassion and concern for the person but the acknowledgement of my clinical skills felt like a welcome boost to my own flagging confidence.

At the end of this time, I noticed a poster on the wall in the staff room. It was an invitation for psychiatry registrars to participate in the Inaugural Australasian Psychiatry Essay Competition, sponsored by the journal, Australasian Psychiatry. The topic for the essay was a quote from the well-known Australian psychiatrist John Ellard.

Although science is an essential part of psychiatry, it is not its essence.

I knew the moment I read that quote that I had to write the essay. All the writing and thinking I had been doing in the years prior to this invitation had equipped me to have some meaningful things to say about why science is essential, and yet is not the essence of psychiatry. The most important experience I had so far been exposed to in terms of the essence of psychiatry was the humanity of Tony Ryle's approach to me when I was young. It was the quality of the relationship we were able to develop that had made such a difference. Even though it didn't protect me from further extreme states, this experience, and my own recovery, essentially guided my clinical work. I was also aware, however, how important it was to be able to do good research in order to demonstrate the effectiveness of an intervention.

The essay virtually wrote itself. I expounded the importance of the scientific method and of asking the right questions in order to find helpful answers in psychiatry. I reflected on the importance of the 'connexional' dimension of human experience, and the need for the people practising psychiatry to have the capacity to develop meaningful human connection with the people we serve. Putting forward my view that the essence of psychiatry lay in the quality of the relationship between 'doctor' and 'patient', I also mentioned the issue of worldview and spirituality.

Once it was written, I somehow 'knew' that it would win the essay competition. I was about to start my next training job, so I read the essay to Dr Sandy Simpson, my new supervisor, and told him what happened to me. As I was posting the essay, I had a strange notion that I would hear the result on my birthday. After several months, during which I had been really enjoying working on the forensic unit with Sandy, my birthday came. I still had not heard anything. I could not resist the temptation to call the college in Australia before the end of the day to ask what was happening.

'Well, Dr Randal, I can't let you know just yet, but I can tell you that the winner has been chosen and we will be announcing the results tomorrow. Let me just say that you have nothing to worry about'.

I always felt as if I won that competition on my birthday, but really it was the next day when I heard that I was the winner. The essay was published in Australasian Psychiatry in December 1995, with the title *Divining Psychiatry* (Randal, 1995). The front cover of the journal had a picture of ripples flowing out in circles on the surface of a pool of water, with the caption: 'Psychiatry: What is its essence?'

The editorial noted that four of the five judges had independently put my essay in first place and the fifth had it in second place, with a joke about the scientific, statistical significance of the results. The editor went on to mention that all three winning essays were from New Zealand and wrote: 'The future of New Zealand psychiatry appears to be in good hands'.

When I read this comment, I recalled with a smile the words that the professor had written in his 1989 letter, telling me that I would not be reappointed as a registrar.

> there has been persistent concern amongst your supervisors that your ideas and theoretical models of psychiatry differ significantly from theirs and from what is considered to be standard practice, in such a way as to raise questions about your ability to practise psychiatry in accordance with what we perceive as New Zealand's needs.

It was a pinnacle experience. I was vindicated. If my life ended at that point, it would have been worth it. God sure does work in mysterious ways. Looking back now, it was such a poignant irony after what had happened to me.

106

Although I was still far from a position in which New Zealand psychiatry might be considered as in any way being 'in my hands', I felt encouraged to proceed with my ongoing training. In the meantime, I was having some healing experiences working with forensic patients, under Sandy Simpson's guidance. Like me, and unlike most psychiatrists both at that time and now, he was interested in the rehabilitation of people with severe and enduring psychotic states. He was supportive of my work. He was also compassionate and understanding towards me. I often cried in the context of supervision, as I reflected on the painful journey I had experienced in psychiatry. One of the things Tony Ryle had said to me all those years ago was that I needed to grieve. The tears, that had been a long time coming, were healing and necessary.

I gained such a lot during my time working in the secure unit. Together with winning the essay competition, it did wonders for my damaged confidence. I was working alongside people who had killed or harmed others or been dangerous in serious ways, often when psychotic. This proved demanding but also rewarding. Finding avenues to connect and communicate meaningfully with them in such a way as to help bring insight and a desire for self-responsibility was fulfilling. I learned to use many different pathways towards connecting with people, depending on what mattered most to them.

After I left the forensic unit, there were a few people I continued to see, each for around 200 sessions. In contrast to their previous lack of progress, they did well after I began working with them. This was apparent in improved scores on standardised assessments and reports from their families and from staff. Like the case with acupuncturists in my doctoral research, it was clear to me that what I was doing worked. I wanted to be able to demonstrate that this was a repeatable effect in other settings. Maybe it would be possible, after all, to set up the research project that I had envisioned for so long.

In the afterglow of these events, I wrote up the 'case histories' required for completion of the psychiatry exams and sat my written papers. In my smart black dress and a sparkling necklace, I went to the college conference in Wellington to collect my prize for winning the essay competition. It was a wonderful feeling!

I found out that I had passed my written exams and case histories with high grades. The next step was the clinical finals which would complete my fellowship exams prior to becoming a senior registrar, and then a consultant psychiatrist. To pass these, we had an hour in a room with a patient, not observed. We then had 20 minutes to organise our thoughts before presenting the person's story – our understanding of them, diagnosis, and treatment plan – to the examiners. It was everything I hated about psychiatry. This was the focus of our training. It was nothing to do with being with the person. The exam failure rate was high, but the consultants I was practising with were encouraging that I was on track to pass.

Because of the long break in my training due to having been ejected, I knew I was at a disadvantage. Two weeks before my clinical exams were scheduled,

I contracted an influenza virus and became severely physically unwell. I was only just recovering when I sat the exams. Cam flew down with me, while our children stayed behind in Auckland with friends. During the clinical exam, my heart was racing, and there was a weight on my chest. Breathing deeply was not an option. One of the people I had to assess was a woman with anorexia. There was no Eating Disorders registrar run in Auckland, and I knew little about this condition. The second case was a man who told me he was feeling acutely suicidal that day, and I felt I had to be with him in a way that was helpful for him, rather than focus on the exam.

Late that afternoon I was told that I had failed.

That news was devastating. To have come so far, only to fail to achieve my goal once more! Once again, I was in a situation where the circumstances were overwhelming and unbearable. That evening we had dinner with friends. They were supportive as I shed a few tears, but it was hard for me to sleep that night. In retrospect I can see that I was on the verge of re-covering the old ground of vulnerability to a massive stress that I could not process. I might so easily have experienced another extreme state. But thankfully – I didn't.

In those days when I woke up in the mornings, I had a daily routine of reading from a Christian book called *Living Light*. The morning after I had failed the exam, the first words of the reading for that day said:

> I myself will go with you and give you success. Be strong! Be courageous! Do not be afraid of them! For the Lord your God will be with you. He will *never fail you* nor forsake you.

It felt to me in that moment as if God had shown up once again at a crucial time and spoken to me in person. Suddenly I felt calm and confident. I could breathe. The fact that the college had failed me was insignificant in comparison with the promise that God would *never* fail me. I recalled that I was under God's authority, the authority of Love and not under the authority of the College of Psychiatry or the Auckland psychiatry training scheme. I felt totally trusting and a sense of deep peace.

Although I could not meaningfully share this with Cam, I held those words in my heart as we travelled back to Auckland. We had arranged to go on a six-week trip to England, Europe, and America to visit my family and friends following my exams, and I was able to enjoy that trip wholeheartedly. We took our two boys, who were by now aged 10 and 14, and met up with my oldest son who was 22 years old and working in France. We had a truly magical time, culminating in a wonderful trip to Disneyland on the way back.

On my return to work, I began a registrar run at Buchanan Clinic, a 36-bed, inpatient medium-and-long-stay mental health unit set up in the early nineties during the closure of Carrington Hospital, the psychiatric hospital where I had begun my training in the mid-eighties. It was for those people who were unable to be rehomed in the community because of their high level of need for care. I was delighted to be working with Dr Debbie Antcliff once again, as I had so enjoyed her consultant oversight almost a decade earlier.

I intended to re-sit the clinical final exam within the year. It was almost universal that Auckland psychiatry registrars in those days would fail at least one attempt at the clinicals, and most passed on the second or third attempt. I began to form supportive and healing relationships with the people I was serving. As the registrar, it was my duty to get to know all the people who lived at the hospital to some extent, although I was mainly involved with the younger people in the shorter stay unit.

Then, almost at the end of the run, in the summer of 1996, Debbie told me that she was going to be taking six weeks leave. She expressed confidence in my clinical abilities and was happy to leave me in charge of the hospital in her absence. I felt encouraged by her belief in me and took up the challenge with a sense of excitement. I knew that once I passed my clinical exams, I would be in a position of leadership and responsibility as a senior registrar, and later as a psychiatrist. This was a good opportunity to practise. Usually, of course, there would be a consultant plus a registrar covering the hospital, and while Debbie was away, I would be on my own, but I would have the oversight of the local Clinical Director of Psychiatry at the District Health Board.

Everything went well for the first month of Debbie's leave. The staff seemed happy with my leadership style, and the people we served seemed to be remarkably settled with their care and support. However, it was brought to my attention that staff were noticing erratic behaviour in a colleague, and that her breath smelt of alcohol in the mornings. The situation was particularly complicated by the fact that she had been working on the acute ward in the main hospital when I had been admitted there overnight all those years before in the aftermath of the interview with the two professors. I was able to discuss the situation with the clinical director and received the support I needed to manage it appropriately.

Then a second difficult personal conundrum arose. A young woman, who coincidentally had also been on the acute ward when I was a patient for that one night, was readmitted to the long-stay ward. She recognised me and refused to be 'treated by someone with a mental illness'. Again, I was able to access the support of the clinical director. Debbie was due to return shortly anyway, and the other staff were familiar with this young woman so my role for her at that time was minimal.

A third challenge was not so easily negotiated. There was a young man on the unit with whom I felt I had a good therapeutic alliance as his doctor. He was beginning to open up and tell me about some aspects of his childhood that had been traumatic for him. Then one morning a male staff member, with whom I also had a good working relationship, told me confidentially that this young man was making accusations that I had looked at him in a 'sexual' way.

My heart sank. I was worried that I might have done something that might have harmed him. I flicked through my memories of our interactions. Had I been too warm towards him, or mis-attuned to his needs? I was very shocked. It seemed likely that my empathic listening must have been misinterpreted in the aftermath of his prior experiences. My immediate response was, as always, to contact the clinical director, and this time to include a call to my Medical Defence Union, and to submit an incident form.

We were able to address the young man's concerns in a way that was apparently beneficial for him, as he was taken seriously. His needs were met appropriately and effectively by the excellent staff on the unit. However, for me, this was the final straw. I stopped sleeping and that familiar heavy pressure settled on my chest. The agitation was so intense I could hardly keep still.

I consulted the clinical director, asking for sick leave even though Debbie wouldn't be back for a week. He listened supportively and tried to help me figure out what had happened. My fear was not only that I had done some terrible harm, but also that I would be crucified for it. The events might have unleashed the Pandora's box of shame about making mistakes that I had grappled with almost all my life. I felt protected by the clinical director's reassurance that I had done nothing wrong. However, within 24 hours after leaving work, I was catapulted into yet another extreme state.

I have little detail in my memory of the content this time.

I am pacing round and round the house, noticing patterned arrangements everywhere. I am unable to decipher their meaning. I 'see' newspaper photos moving as if they are being projected onto mini television sets.

My own private psychiatrist was away on holiday at the time and not contactable. One of my close friends, who was by now a qualified psychiatrist, came and stayed the night. Another psychiatrist, a senior colleague who had supervised my clinical work during my break in training, visited me the next day. The support they so generously offered meant I did not end up back in the acute ward. He and my friend persuaded me to take risperidone, which was a new 'antipsychotic' that was marketed as very safe and effective.

I am thinking that this drug will probably kill me, but I am prepared to take it for the sake of my family – and to die if need be.

Fortunately, I didn't die. I went to see my psychiatrist as soon as she returned. By then, I was more or less back to my rational self, although once again shaken and unhappy. Thankfully, as with previous times, the acute altered state of consciousness only lasted a few days, but my behaviour was clearly upsetting for everyone. My oldest son had found my extreme states intolerable years before, when he was a teenager. He had made the wise decision to live with his father in America, a sad choice for me at the time. I did not want to put my younger sons or Cam through any more turmoil and pain. I wanted to be a good wife, and a good parent. I also wanted to be a good patient and to make everything better for everyone. If necessary, I was prepared to take medication on a regular basis for the rest of my life in the hope that it would prevent ever having another episode.

Debbie came to see me at home with a bright bunch of flowers when she returned from her leave. She expressed her concern and care, telling me to take as much time off as I needed, but to get back to work when I was ready. It was quite remarkable to see how supportive everyone had become towards enabling me to continue in my career in psychiatry. This was despite the now obvious fact that stressors, including work stressors, could potentially destabilise my mental health. No one could be accused of repeating the crime of stigma and discrimination that had been enacted against me in the past. The stigmatisation that was happening now was self-stigmatisation. Once again, I gradually became less self-confident and struggled to maintain a sense of direction and purpose. It did not seem a good idea to re-sit my clinical finals. I felt diminished. I decided to take myself out of the psychiatry training scheme; I didn't want to become a consultant psychiatrist after all.

Over the years since leaving England, I had tried seeing a number of different therapists. Nothing had been effective in stopping these episodes. I began to take on the devastating, spirit-breaking notion that I was going to continue to have recurrent bouts of psychosis. Cam and I felt that it would be best if I continued taking a small dose of risperidone from then on. It's as if I took on the role of doctoring myself. But in the back of my mind, there was the echo of the words from the day after my failed attempt at my clinical exams: 'I will never fail you or forsake you. I will go with you and give you success'.

JOSEPHINE'S STORY 1985–1995
(AGES 31–41)

14

AFTER AFRICA
Rekindling Passion for Medicine and Love

In which Josephine grapples with the demands of the doctor role, learns more about loving and being loved and finds a pathway to committed service.

Returning to life as a house surgeon felt strange after my time in Africa. I experienced a kind of imposter syndrome, stunned when I expressed an opinion about what should be done and people followed my instructions. My impulse was to say, 'It's only me!' It was still the days of working 13 days in a row and 56-hour weekends on call. Wandering around the hospital on a Monday afternoon, often having had little sleep since Saturday morning, I was desperate to get home. But being so exhausted, I was struggling to focus my mind to get through the list of tasks I had to complete before I left. The house officer years were a lonely, desolate time, feeling physically and mentally spent, and not knowing if I would ever find a life partner.

The challenges of finding my place as a person, and a doctor in my role with patients, faded into the background. Survival was my primary focus. But one important and different memory, which I struggled to process at the time, still guides my practice. The patient was a severely ill woman in her 70s, who was dependent on significant medical intervention to keep her alive. Her husband didn't seem to realise this and was begging the physician to let her go home. As part of the flock of doctors around her bed, observing this conversation in a ward, I felt impatient with the consultant. I wanted to move on. He wasn't making it clear that discharging her was not an option; she would die without hospital care. To my astonishment, the physician agreed to her discharge. She didn't deteriorate into death. Against all expectations she improved at home. I feel emotional as I write this. That physician was a powerful model for me in his recognition of the wisdom of the family, and that doctors don't know everything.

A bright spot towards the end of this period, which developed into a shining star over my life, is that Ian and I got back together and married. We had lived apart for six years – painful years for both of us – but once we were together

DOI: 10.4324/9781003153788-21

again, we never looked back. It wasn't until the process of writing this book that I have come to have some understanding of why I left the man I loved all those years before.

In my childhood, I had developed a belief that I had to appear happy for people who were important to me. It felt vital to me that I did not need or depend on them. My falling in love with Ian was partly because he did not need that from me. When we first met, I thrived in the relationship with him, feeling loved and cared for, and we had a lot of good times. To allow myself to be vulnerable and nurtured by Ian was new and exciting; I was happy in the relationship. However, my early conditioning that I should not need anything from people close to me would not allow me to settle in this relationship. I felt that to grow up I had to be independent and manage without this kind of care. Returning to the relationship had not seemed an option until – I don't know how – I gradually became free within myself to connect with Ian again. Thank goodness. We have three wonderful children and have lived happily ever after, more or less. Getting some clarity on this process has increased the depth of connection I have with Ian now.

I still had no great passion for medicine and had seen myself as working part-time as a family doctor while I had children. The idea of entering specialist training with years more of working through the clock, and having to use all my spare time to study, made me shudder. However, things changed after watching the movie, *The Killing Fields*. This told the story of the atrocities under the Pol Pot regime in Cambodia. Feeling overwhelmed by the suffering it depicted, I felt compelled to enter the field of medicine where I had the most contribution to make. This was psychiatry. Perhaps I had not totally lost my sense of the people inside the bodies we were treating. This was a full circle back to my decision at age 15 – to focus on non-physical aspects of people's well-being.

15

FEELING LOST IN PSYCHIATRY AND FOUND IN MOTHERING

In which Josephine has contrasting experiences in being a psychiatry registrar and being a mother in terms of both offering and receiving care and support.

Like Patte, I was astounded to find so little psychotherapeutic input in the acute psychiatric hospitals. Through Youthline, I had done training in talking therapies and was keen to do more. I was disappointed. The approach was almost totally biological and custodial. One psychological strategy, used when family relationships were identified as a problem, was described as a 'parentectomy' – meaning a kind of 'operation' to remove parents. Instead of going home, alternative accommodation was found for the young person in a boarding house. At the time I wasn't familiar with these boarding houses and didn't know what a bleak existence they could be. Even so I found this approach incomprehensible. But I didn't challenge it.

One day, as a psychiatry registrar, I was sitting in an assessment with a psychiatrist talking with a woman who was visibly distressed. My instinct was to reach out to her and offer some comfort. However, I realised that this was not acceptable. My role was to sit and observe, collecting data which would enable us to make the correct diagnosis and prescribe the most effective treatment. Unlike Patte, I allowed myself to be controlled by these prohibitions on engaging with patients on a human level. I applied myself to building my skills and focusing my listening on identifying indicators of illness in order to establish a *diagnosis* rather than listening for understanding. I came to the somewhat cynical conclusion that a psychiatric interview was a way of having a conversation with someone in an extreme state, in significant distress, without being with them in any meaningful way.

Had I met Patte in her first extreme state, I would have thought I knew just what to do. Compulsory containment using the Mental Health Act would have seemed necessary because of the level of disorganisation and risk (jumping off the top of the stairs). I would have identified an elevated or labile mood (high or rapidly changing emotional state). I would have listened to the

DOI: 10.4324/9781003153788-22

experiences of being in the vanguard of a transformational movement, and pulling people into a new reality. I would have identified these ideas as 'grandiose'. This would contribute towards a diagnosis of mania. I would also have identified her running through the campus hugging people and entering Tony's room when he was seeing someone else, as an increased level of activity and loss of usual social inhibitions. This would further support the diagnosis of mania. I would have prescribed 'antipsychotic' medication. In those days we might even have locked her in a seclusion room and given her 100 mg of chlorpromazine an hour until she went to sleep. Given Patte's response to chlorpromazine, we might even have killed her!

I would have wanted more information about her sleep. I would have asked how she had been functioning in the days, weeks, and months before this event. I might have sought a developmental history. My work in psychiatry happened a decade or so later than this event and I was aware of the significance of trauma for people by then, so I might have asked about it. But I would have seen it as another issue, along with the grief for her father and the babies who died, to be addressed when the psychosis had been treated with medication.

I would not have listened to the *content* of what Patte was saying or looked for meaning related to her experiences. I would not have made the connection that violation of trust is a key issue with sexual abuse and that trust is a key in the extreme experience. I would not have wondered about a connection between forgetting in the extreme-state experience of forgetting and her mother having asked her to forget the sexual abuse. I would not have wondered if the idea that 'we are all the same' was an attempt by her mind to let Patte off the hook of the superhuman expectations she developed for herself quite early in her childhood. Had I met her again in another extreme state, I may well have diagnosed Bipolar Disorder and recommended that she stay on long-term medication. I would have missed Patte as a person.

In my early work in the acute wards, it was painful for me to watch people caught in vicious cycles in the emotionally intense, unstable environments there. Watching their spirits being broken and feeling unable to contribute, when I was part of the institution that was damaging them, was perplexing and demoralising for me. Some good feedback came my way, but I tended to find it mystifying.

We used much larger doses of sedating and antipsychotic medication in those days. Even at that time, I could see that though these medications were calming, they also dulled people's senses and intellect. A couple of people stood out in my mind as particularly trapped. They would respond to emotional intensity around them with increased emotional instability, agitation, and sometimes aggression. We then increased restrictions on their freedom and increased doses of sedating medication. It was hard to see how they could get out of this vicious cycle. Then I realised that the long-stay wards could be an opportunity for them to get away from the chaotic environment that had been so triggering for them. It underlines what a dearth of options we had, that long-stay wards seemed a therapeutic possibility. Initially I couldn't get anyone to listen to me. The people caught in these cycles did not fit the criteria for the long-stay wards. But my battling was fuelled by the frustration, powerlessness, and vicarious pain I felt for all the people for whom I could do so little. Finally, the rules were bent, and they were able to move. Their lives were not transformed, but at least they shifted a little.

I was shocked by the tendency to blame families and I did my best to engage with them. When I was in the hospital on call, I sometimes met with families in the evening. One night I was feeling particularly stuck. My bleeper sounded and I left the room, grateful for the interruption. It was my mother, ringing for a social chat. When I told her that I was struggling with a family, she gave me simple instructions:

Ask each member of the family in turn how they see the challenges, what they have tried and what they have noticed.

If you find the conversation is getting stuck or derailed, then ask one member of the family to describe what they thought the feelings or thoughts of another member of the family would be.

Following her advice seemed to help the conversation go better. The young man's mother was particularly appreciative when he left the hospital. I used these simple strategies a lot. They enabled a different sort of conversation, with more explicit communication and some increased understanding of each other. Families grappling with the emotional roller coaster of being involved with an acute psychiatric unit seemed to find this helpful.

On another night on call I realised my efforts to connect with the people I was trying to serve may have been more effective than I thought. The police brought in a man I had met on previous admissions. He was physically large with a criminal and drug-use history and a diagnosis of Bipolar Disorder. He was intoxicated, disorganised, irritable, and assaultive. The staff were in the process of restraining and sedating him when I appeared. They paused so I could assess him. He made eye contact with me and slowed down a bit. He was able to regulate himself by engaging in conversation with me as a familiar person. It touched my heart to feel I was of some use to someone.

The therapy approaches I had learned – Rogerian counselling, Solution Focused Therapy and Narrative Therapy – were not valued in psychiatry. Psychodynamic psychotherapy was the approach understood as valid therapy for non-psychotic people. This is despite the lack of evidence base at the time. The psychodynamic psychotherapy, which was so valued, operated from an expert based approach. The clinician would question and listen to the patient while developing hypotheses as to why they were functioning in the way they were. Explanations were usually deficit-based, with considerable weight given to the role of damaging early life experiences. A significant therapeutic intervention was for the therapist to explain what was happening for them. The hierarchical nature of the approach was neither congruent with the values I had been brought up with, nor the therapeutic approaches I had encountered. In my enthusiasm to excel in the world of psychiatry, I tried to let go what I had previously learned and valued, and to apply myself to learning psychodynamic psychotherapy.

When I was allocated to work in one of only two psychotherapeutically oriented programmes in Auckland, I was excited. Now, perhaps, I could learn to engage with people in a way which made a difference for them. Despite all my efforts to suppress my discomfort and fit myself to their models, my alternative and, in this context, anti-establishment, ideas must have leaked out in a way that was uncomfortable for the programme leaders. I experienced a systematic invalidation of myself and my judgement.

An example of this happened with a young person I had met on previous admissions to the acute wards, who I will call Alex. Alex had a mood disorder with episodes of psychosis. After my assessment, I presented my opinion to the team that this programme would not be suitable for Alex because the level of interpersonal challenge might pose a risk of causing decompensation into psychosis. My opinion was overruled, and Alex came in to the programme. I told myself I must have been wrong in my assessment.

In conversation with me on my own one day, Alex spoke about extreme experiences which I understood as delusions, or part of a psychosis. When I reported this back to the team, the conclusion was that I was bringing this forward in order to support my earlier view and establish my place in the team as an expert in illness, as I clearly was not an expert in psychotherapy. I felt chastened. Alex decompensated into psychosis a few days later and was transferred back to the acute unit. I still wonder if there might have been a way I could have used my observations to prevent this. If *I* had developed psychosis after this I would have understood why. I didn't, but felt demolished as a clinician. I lost confidence, not only in my judgement, but also in my sense that I had something to offer clinically as a person.

This experience did not decrease my determination to develop expertise in psychodynamic psychotherapy. I thought I just had to try harder. Throughout my training, I attended night classes, organised psychodynamic supervision for myself and had three attempts at engaging in my own therapy. But it was a fraught pathway for me. In several of these learning situations, I ended up in conflicts reminiscent of the conflicts I'd had early in secondary school; feeling judged by someone in power for doing what felt like being myself.

At the end of this psychotherapy run I went on maternity leave. I felt driven to have a baby with what felt like a biological urge. But I was terrified of losing my identity as a career woman. I felt I was at risk of 'suburban neurosis', a sort of depressed state some women experience, feeling trapped and isolated in homes, tending to young children. No one had paternity leave in those days. When Ian returned to work a few days after I had my first baby,

I had no idea how I would get through the day. I was so wrong. Nothing prepared me for how much I delighted in having children. Both Ian and I were overwhelmed with the love we felt.

For the birth of my first baby, I went into hospital for only a few hours and left as soon as I could. A midwife who had done lots of home births supported me through the first ten days at home. She seemed very tuned-in and responsive. There was a story that a baby had died during delivery in the local specialist hospital. Apparently, the baby was hooked up to a monitor but no one was looking at the monitor. It seemed to me that I was better off with the quality attention of this attuned, experienced midwife at home than being in hospital with all the medical expertise. My second and third children were born at home supported by this same midwife.

As a new mother, I turned into a breastfeeding blancmange. I managed, but 'down functioned'. For about nine years, I didn't work more than half time, sometimes not at all, sometimes as little as two days a week. I was there for my children but no one would have called me a super-mum. Embracing the life of a mum at home, I took the children to Playcentre, a cooperative preschool where parents stay with their children. It felt an extraordinary privilege for me and my children to be part of a community focused around cooperatively supporting our children to flourish. Lifelong friendships developed, for the children and for Ian and me.

Despite the tiredness, and feeling as ground down as I ever had as a house officer, there were so many peak experiences. A five-year-old mastering the use of a diving mask underwater, looking up at me and exclaiming with joy, 'I can see your legs'. Skiing downhill with a child between my legs. Finding I had the courage to defend my two-year-old from an aggressive goose wanting the bread we were trying to feed to the ducks. Watching my five-year-old jumping out of the car for school, running to catch up with his older sisters, not a thought for me. I could go on and on.

When I worked two days a week, too little to be in the training scheme or be on the afterhours roster, these were precious times. Most of my world was pre-schoolers, but I also had a toe in the psychiatry world. Managing, as a mother, to meet the needs of my children stretched me, but in the Playcentre context, I felt no pressure to appear to manage. We were all struggling together. This enabled me to do some important unlearning about how to be superhuman and to learn to depend on Ian.

16

BEGINNING TO FIND MY PLACE
IN PSYCHIATRY

In which Josephine experiences contrasting practices inside and
outside institutional psychiatry and begins to see a pathway for
positive change in her practice of psychiatry.

Pre-schoolers were the centre of my world, but I continued to plod through
my psychiatry training. After the period in the psychotherapy unit, when I'd
felt demolished as a clinician, I stopped work to have my first baby and went
back part-time. Having lost confidence in my clinical judgement made it difficult for me to work effectively. Apparently my first supervisor expressed
concerns about the quality of my work, although I do not remember this
being discussed with me. In my next run, I was doing a presentation to the
grand round, a frightening prospect. It was not a supportive collaborative learning environment but a battleground where academic psychiatrists
engaged in competitive sparring. On the morning I was to do my presentation, I received a letter from the head of the training scheme to say that if
I did not pull my socks up, I would be out of the programme. No one had
approached me to ask me how I was finding work, or to try and understand
what might be happening.

After reading this letter, I continued with my morning's work and presented
my talk. It was on the phenomenology of affect (emotions people show) in
psychotic illness. As I had with so many other challenges, I managed. I got
through creditably until the director of the training scheme asked about
treatment. When I said that was outside the scope of the talk, he asked disparagingly, 'What was the point of doing a presentation which did not address
treatment?' It was all I could do to continue standing on the platform without
dissolving into tears. The rest of the session went by in a blur. He came up
to me afterwards to tell me what a good talk it was, and to admonish me for
not using the good brain I apparently had, in my work. If my spirit was not
broken, it was significantly injured.

The added identity I had as a mother was crucial to maintaining my sanity
through my training. In retrospect, I realise it also provided invaluable life

DOI: 10.4324/9781003153788-23

experiences. One of these was the experience of engaging with the world as fat. When I was breastfeeding, my body generated hunger for more food than I needed. The only way I could have not put on weight would have been to feel hungry most of the time. Engaging with the world as 'fat' is significantly less enjoyable than engaging with the world as 'not fat'. It was not so bad for me, valued and well connected in my family, work, and social worlds. It was also time limited. But inflicting unwanted weight gain on young people with psychotic illnesses as a result of the antipsychotic medication they have no choice but to take is another matter. One of the effects of psychosis is loss of motivation and finding it harder to engage socially. To have the burden of obesity added to these struggles seemed almost too cruel.

There was little information available about this weight gain associated with anti-psychotic medication. Supported by my old friend, Bruce Arroll, and my longing to find some way of contributing to people's lives, I read everything I could find and wrote a literature review. It was well received when I presented it at a psychiatry conference, and later it was accepted for publication (Stanton, 1995). This reconnecting with my academic self also helped me move towards feeling I had something to offer.

There were two psychiatrists who were particularly helpful in enabling me to rebuild some of the confidence I needed to be of any real use to people. Both of them operated outside the training scheme, not usually supervising registrars. Both were somewhat counter-cultural in the way they worked.

One was Bill Rowntree. He had a chequered history, but he helped me. He supervised my long psychotherapy case. It was a requirement for psychiatry registrars to see a patient for at least 50 sessions. When I was asked if I would see a particular patient, I found it hard to believe that anyone would think I could have something to offer. It was impossible for me to question the wisdom of the referral. Had I had some clinical confidence, I would have agreed to check the person out, begun with a formal assessment and concluded that the range of issues she was experiencing was too complex and challenging for a junior trainee. However, in my lifelong pattern of not letting anyone, including myself, see my fears I might not be able to manage, I just began.

This whole situation could have become another vicious cycle, for her and for me, had I had a different sort of supervisor who continued to pathologise me. I could have lost further confidence and become increasingly ineffective in my work which would also not have been helpful for the woman. But Bill was able to support me to 'be with' her. In one supervision conversation, where I was feeling particularly out of my depth, he gave me some simple, practical advice.

'Just repeat the last few words of each sentence she says'.

Restricting myself rigidly from doing this felt rather mechanical but she didn't seem to notice. Our sessions became unstuck. We both survived and I learned a lot. I hope she had some benefit.

The other psychiatrist whose influence made a difference for me was Fraser McDonald. My mother had talked about him when I was about 11. In the 1960s, there was a ward in an old psychiatric hospital for mentally disabled children not able to be cared for anywhere else. Their behaviour was out of control. People hated working there and so they could not recruit and retain staff. There were never enough workers, and children were not getting adequate care. Increasing their unmanageable behaviour was the only strategy they could manifest to get the attention they so desperately needed. Negative attention is better than none. Fraser had the idea of engaging well-resourced housewives, including my mother, to come in at mealtimes to feed these children. I remember her shuddering with revulsion at the repulsive behaviour of the child she was feeding. I don't know what she saw but I had a vision of a naked, deformed child smearing food. However, like the other housewives who volunteered there, she drew on her competence and experience in feeding children. The children's behaviour changed. The care these women were able to offer was part of what enabled staff to interrupt the apparently hopeless vicious cycle the children were caught in.

At the time I worked with him, Fraser held a pivotal role in Odyssey House, a structured therapeutic community for rehabilitation of people with drug addiction who often had criminal histories. Many of the staff were recovering addicts themselves. Their lived experience was crucial to the programme. Fraser suggested that I lead the parents' group there. He spoke to me about my lived experience, my knowledge, and skills as a parent, and how this is what I would offer. It worked. I was able to be effective in running a parents' group. He died while still working there, leaving a huge gap. I then took up the clinical role left by his absence.

Initially I was afraid that I would be experienced as second best to Fraser, which would have been an accurate assessment. But it was not like that. I felt appreciated for who I was and what I offered. This was an uplifting place to work. At least in part, this was due to the role of recovering addicts on the staff. It was hard to sit in a staff meeting and feel judgemental of a new person coming in who had assaulted, cheated, lied, and stolen in the grips of their addiction, when the staff member you were sitting next to may well have had a similar history. By extension, I was able to let go of some of my own self-judging.

17

JUMPING THROUGH HOOPS AND BECOMING A PATIENT

In which Josephine confronts some challenges in the rituals and practices of institutional psychiatry.

For many years, I could not face the idea of giving up my lifestyle and devoting all my spare energy to preparing for exams. But once my third child was born, I suddenly developed the drive I needed. Studying was challenging with three pre-schoolers, but I studied whenever they slept. I used to dictate what I needed to learn onto cassettes, take the children walking in the push-chair and watch them play in playgrounds while I listened to the cassettes on a Walkman. I hope they weren't scarred by the limited quality of this attention. Ian was also hugely supportive, even taking our three young children away for weekends – not a small task at the end of a working week.

On the morning of the second written exam, I was unable to stop crying. Initially, I could not process my feeling; it was not anxiety. Then I realised it was humiliation. I was jumping through a hoop. It felt as if I would be defined as satisfactory or a failure, depending on how much rapid focused writing I could do in the upcoming three hours.

Fortunately, I passed. This meant I could sit the clinical exam in Adelaide six weeks later. My chance of passing was limited as I was under-prepared, but I decided to take that chance. Even if I failed, the experience would at least increase the likelihood of passing at my next attempt. I failed. The fail was much more painful than I expected. Few people passed those specialist exams without at least one fail. Despite this, I felt shame. I found it hard to speak about it to colleagues. It took all my self-discipline to get myself back into the process of practising for the next sitting.

As a mother at home working hard to parent three young children, it had felt like a break to shut myself up in a room with books. But preparing for the oral was quite different. It involved an endless process of asking people for favours, patients to practise with and psychiatrists and physicians to act as examiners. I had to make myself available to meet their convenience as well as do my half time job and care for the children. Rushing around between

DOI: 10.4324/9781003153788-24

hospitals and clinics, it seemed inevitable that sooner or later I would be involved in a car accident. When it happened and I was not hurt, I just sat in my car feeling so grateful. Ian was rather cross when I came home with no details about the car that had hit me. I just felt glad to be alive. At the next sitting, I passed the exam. It was great to pass but it felt more like stopping hitting my head against a brick wall than a cause for joy.

Passing this exam took three years of focused study – memorising from psychiatry texts and journals, and honing skills in demonstrating to examiners my ability to assess and develop a treatment plan based on a 50-minute interview. My friend worked as a counsellor. During this time, she was engaging with people, finding ways to improve their lives, searching out the most skilled supervisors, and taking up training opportunities in the most recent developments in therapeutic approaches. I felt envious.

Beaten around by the exam process, I could not seem to recover my energy and zest for life. I decided antidepressants might help, so I went to my family doctor for a prescription. Like Patte, I was doctoring myself. When I first wrote about this, I described not really having a depression, just having some depressive symptoms. Reviewing it I thought, is this me, as a psychiatrist self-stigmatising, identifying a diagnosis of depression as something other people have, and I don't? Prior to doing our study, I had read several papers reporting research about doctors with depressive and anxiety symptoms, but not much about doctors with diagnoses of depression and anxiety disorders. Are diagnoses something for the people we treat but not for us? If I didn't have a diagnosis of depression, what was I doing taking antidepressants? The stressors leading to my symptoms were obvious. Was I more invested in pharmaceutical approaches than I wanted to admit? Was I so entrenched in my reluctance to acknowledge vulnerability that I would take medication but not explore other avenues? This episode, which I initially described as a flirtation with psychiatric medication and diagnosis, is one of the few things I have always been very private about. It's no wonder the consultation with my doctor felt uncomfortable. Added to all this, I couldn't stop myself assessing the job she was doing in assessing me for depression!

I stopped taking the antidepressants because I lost my interest in sex which is a documented side effect. My generous husband had been through enough! I threw myself into a new project of finding our family the house for the rest of our lives. My energy (and interest in sex) came back. When we bought a house that we couldn't afford, some of my friends worried that I was having a manic episode! I opened a private practice on Thursday evenings and Saturday mornings, and leapt into the next phase of my life.

There were a couple of other notable occasions when I took my doctor self into the patient role. In these instances, I saw my doctor and had a sort of collegial chat but failed to communicate my suffering. The first time was when I had mastitis (infected milk ducts) when my third child was a few weeks old. I was barely able to walk to the bathroom. Friends had taken the other children. Ian put water in baby bottles for me as I felt too weak to sit up to drink. He went to work, planning to come back at lunchtime to help me go to the bathroom and change the baby. The front door was left open so the doctor could get in. I lay in bed, sipping the water and intermittently breastfeeding my baby. The doctor came, examined me in bed and conferred with me about the diagnosis of mastitis, asking me what I thought. What I *thought*? I could hardly hold my eyes open and look at him; I couldn't think, let alone talk intelligently. I just wanted help! I suspect that he had no idea how sick I was. I didn't tell him.

Some years later I had a brief episode of an autoimmune disorder with intensely itchy legs. I hate mosquito bites, but this was another experience. It reminded me of a man I had seen in my first year as a registrar with itching skin all over his body. He had tried to kill himself by hitting himself on the head with a hammer, and now I could identify with that.

It was winter and I got through the day and night by intermittently immersing my legs in cold water to reduce the blood flow to the skin. When I finally went to the doctor, I joined him with my doctor self to engage energetically in comparing my legs with photos in a dermatology book. He wanted to do a biopsy but did not have time in his busy clinic. We agreed on a diagnosis and I went home with nothing to reduce the itching. When I woke in the night with my legs driving me demented, I plunged them into a bath of cold water. I was glad the doctor hadn't had time to do a biopsy as I would have not been able to get relief in this way with a wound in my leg.

Looking up the diagnosis on the internet I found it recommended oral steroids. The next day at work, I was tempted to ask a colleague to look at my legs and write a script. This is what is known as a 'corridor consultation', common among doctors. It was what I would have probably done prior to our work on the research project on doctors as patients. However, I wanted to do it properly. I rang my doctor, left a message for him to ring back and ask the receptionist to interrupt whatever I was doing to get me to the phone. When he rang back, he asked if he had interrupted something. I said that he hadn't, as I'd been outside between appointments putting my legs in a bucket of cold water. He seemed surprised that my legs were causing me so much discomfort and I realised I had not told him. The oral steroids gave me relief within 24 hours.

Part 3

LEARNING FROM EXPERIENCE

PATTE'S STORY 1996–2020 (AGES 45–69)

18

A HERCULEAN TASK

'Hope and a Future'

In which a dream comes true and Patte enables healing for others
but not herself

By now, I was 45 years old, and I had recovered from six episodes of psychosis. It is only in the process of writing this book and reflecting with Josephine about what happened to me, that I have begun to see more clearly how long it took me to regain my resilience each time. After each episode, I have always remarked that, as usual, I recovered very quickly and was back to my normal self within two weeks. It was certainly the way I saw it, but was that an accurate portrayal?

Initially, my recovery from the episode in 1996, following my brief stint at taking on the in-loco consultant role while Debbie was on holiday, was no different from other times. However, I found myself at a crossroad having to make a huge life decision about how to proceed. It was the worst of times, and yet it was to prove ultimately to be the best of times. I knew that in the immediate future, I no longer wanted to repeat my clinical finals and complete my training as a psychiatrist. But what did I want to do instead? For years, I had believed I had a contribution to make to psychiatry. Maybe it would at last be possible to put into practice the hard-earned skills I had learnt in my late twenties. My research degree, which neither I nor my psychiatry colleagues had really valued up to this point, was about to come to my rescue.

Much of what I had been learning to get me through the psychiatry exams seemed to me to be more harmful than helpful. Rather than focusing on getting as much information as possible from a person in order to formulate a diagnosis and treatment plan, what I had enjoyed most in my work was being with people in ways that brought transformation.

Over the years, spending many hours with people such as Gloria and Clara had taught me a lot about what made a difference to their lives. I had continued to develop this type of approach in the forensic unit and during my first six months at Buchanan Clinic. Many of the people I met suffered severe, long-lasting, and debilitating states, which had not responded to any

DOI: 10.4324/9781003153788-27

of the available 'antipsychotic' medications. They usually had diagnoses of so-called schizophrenia, and often lived in isolation, even when other people were physically nearby. Their realities were frequently determined by voice-hearing experiences or belief systems that were difficult for others to relate to or understand. Being with them in creative, attuned ways came naturally to me and appeared to be making a difference. I wondered whether now might be the time to find out whether the effectiveness of my therapeutic approach could be scientifically validated. When I returned to work a few weeks after my own extreme state had subsided, I had a conversation about this with Debbie and the clinical director of Auckland District Health Board. To my amazement, they gave me the opportunity to change my role at Buchanan Clinic and to take on the official title of 'Research Fellow'. Sandy Simpson agreed to be my research supervisor. I felt grateful for the support they all offered.

After an intense six weeks of reading and writing, I managed to pull together a research protocol. It was extremely hard work. As an underpinning requirement for research, I had to write a literature review and to create a rationale and a framework in which my work could fit. Ethics approval was the next hurdle. Before I knew it, I was training the staff to do the assessments so that the outcomes could be measured. It all happened in such a whirl that I could hardly keep up with myself.

As I got started, the enormity of what I was taking on began to weigh heavily on me. Each day, I woke in the morning feeling anguished. This made absolutely no sense. Researching my own therapeutic approach was something I had longed to do for years. It was a dream come true. Tackling massive projects was my forte. And yet it was all I could do to get myself out of bed, dressed, see to my sons' needs, and get into the car to drive to work. What got me through was knowing others were praying for me, and reminding myself of scriptures I had memorised.

But even with this spiritual support, I was full of mortifying shame and doubt, fearing that everything I was doing would fail to produce any useful outcomes for the people I served, let alone measurable outcomes for my research. Sandy often reminded me that research is always hard to do, especially the sort of intervention research that I was undertaking. He would try to help me see that the cup was half full, but I could only see it as half empty. As the weeks and months unfolded, I assumed that the daily anguish was linked to the sheer effort of keeping up with my commitment to the people in the study, plus the burden of fulfilling my research responsibilities. Nevertheless, I just got on with the task, urged forward by expectations of my own super-humanness, and my sense that this was in some way my destiny.

Sometimes I would try to tell myself that, because my work was important to God, I was under spiritual attack. The raging cosmic battle. A couple of scriptures helped with this. One was from Jeremiah 29:11.

'For I know the plans I have for you', declares the Lord, 'plans to prosper you and not to harm you, plans to give you hope and a future'.

And another was from Isaiah 54:16–17

'And it is I who created the destroyer to wreak havoc; no weapon forged against you will prevail, and you will refute every tongue that accuses you. This is the heritage of the servants of the Lord, and this is their vindication from me'.

Oddly enough, I did not tell my psychiatrist about how hard I was finding each day.

In the narrative that follows, I will describe the type of interaction I had with each of the nine people who agreed to participate in my research. The details of any particular person's experience have been changed to protect the identities of all concerned. At the beginning of the research, all the participants had diagnoses of so-called schizophrenia and schizoaffective disorder and were not making clinical progress over years, despite being on medication considered optimal at the time. Most were taking clozapine, olanzapine, or risperidone. I have combined several stories together and used some fictional examples that capture the essence of the way I worked. Although I was open with my senior colleagues, in those days, I never shared my story with the people I saw therapeutically. It would have seemed entirely unprofessional to me at that time, though my views have since changed. Examples based on my work in the secure setting are mixed in with what I did during my research at Buchanan Clinic. I hope this account remains true to the spirit of what was helpful.

With one woman, I shared books that interested her – usually about her spiritual beliefs, which incidentally were different from mine. We talked about Building a Bridge of Trust, which was a metaphor that came to me somewhere along the way.

'I want to really hear your story; to fully understand what has happened for you and how you see things. I can't promise always to see things in the same way you do, but I certainly can promise that I genuinely want to build that bridge from your reality to mine, so we can come to a shared understanding', I said to her, in one way or another, on several occasions.

She eventually agreed that this sounded worth trying. She felt suspicious of everyone on the ward, and spending time with me meant the occasional outing. At her request, on a couple of occasions, I accompanied her to meet with a spiritual mentor of her choice. Sure enough, the Bridge of Trust gradually got built over time. She began to confide in me her fears that staff could hear her thoughts and were plotting against her.

'What are you noticing that tells you they can hear your thoughts?' I asked her.

'They're often frowning', she said.

'Do you notice that I sometimes frown?'

'Yes', she said. 'You might be in on it too'.

'How about you ask me next time you see me frowning and I promise to tell you what I'm thinking about?' I suggested.

We tried out this strategy for a while. One time I was frowning as I remembered that I had forgotten to take my washing out of the machine before I came to work. Another time I was trying to recall a name I couldn't think of. She would catch me frowning even when I was not aware of it. I had to be prepared to be authentic with her, choosing wisely what to self-disclose. She was prepared to believe me. Over time she became more aware of many other facial expressions, such as when I was smiling. She would ask me why I was smiling, and we would have a dialogue. She began to smile more too. She began to notice that when she smiled at people, they often smiled back. Gradually, she began to wonder whether she was misinterpreting some of the frowning:

'Maybe they forgot their washing too', she joked.

It was a delight to witness her sense of humour. I explained to her about how as doctors we notice the way people think that can be unhelpful, and we give names to these ways of thinking. I told her what the terminology was that we use, so that she could use it too. In some ways, I was breaking new ground and transcending a professional barrier. Rather than being a psychiatrist identifying symptoms, I was sharing this knowledge with her (and went on to do so with others too).

I used the skills I had learnt as a psychiatry registrar as a tool to help her think about her own thinking. For example, thinking people are plotting to harm us because they are frowning can be called an 'idea of reference'. This term is used because a personal meaning is attributed to a behaviour as if it is referring to us, when in reality the frowning could be due to a thousand other reasons. The more she could notice these experiences and name them, the calmer she noticed she felt. She would tell me something about what she was thinking, and then ask, 'Is that an idea of reference?'

Although using different terminology, a similar process later became standard in Cognitive Behavioural Therapy, described as 'identifying thinking errors', but I had not come across this back then.

She began to tell me about the emotions she was having when the upsetting thoughts were most intense. Anxiety and anger were most commonly what she noticed. One day when she was feeling particularly anxious, we tried listening to Abba together in her room, which I knew she enjoyed. I could see that it calmed her down, and she noticed that too. Bit by bit she found ways to manage her distress. By the time my consultant asked her parents about the progress they could recognise in her, I had met with her 173 times. Every minute was worth it, according to her father; she was a changed woman. I was very encouraged by the outcome of this investment of our time, which was a labour of love.

Central to all my work was building a therapeutic alliance, 'being with' each person in whatever way best suited them. I attuned myself to meet their needs for acknowledgement and recognition; in short, being a listening, validating person who genuinely cared for them. My attitude was always one of empathy and compassion. Talking about this as 'building a Bridge of Trust' had been a useful metaphor. I continued to use this image.

Rather than waiting, I would actively seek each person out. I was flexible about time and place, maybe going out for a walk, coffee or a meal, or spending time sitting with them in silence if need be, while they got on with whatever they chose. I spent as much or as little time as they wanted or required. With some people, initially I only spent five or ten minutes being with them, maybe just enough time to say a warm 'hello' and ask if there was anything they might like to do when we next met, and when they would like to get together again. I was always prepared to be spontaneous and change plans if need be, always checking in about how the person was feeling and what would best suit them. Their choice was always paramount as long as it was within the bounds of safety. This may sound very easy and straightforward. From the outside, it could appear that I was doing almost nothing. Yet what was required was careful attention, presence, and attunement. And it was entirely different from the expectations and role of a doctor.

One day, I went to the beach with a young woman. There was little conversation. She had packed her blue swimming togs in a plastic bag, stuffed under a faded, red and yellow beach towel. These were items she was clearly used to grabbing at a moment's notice, and she merrily swung the bag in the crook of her arm, her golden hair lifting and falling gently over her shoulders with every stride towards the sea. I almost had to run to keep up. I am not a swimmer and had only learned to get from one end of the pool to the other a few years earlier. Actually, I was still scared of being out of my depth. I would never choose to go swimming in the sea. She, on the other hand, had been a water baby since childhood. With some trepidation, I waited while she swam out further than I could see. Although the Pohutukawa trees were showing off their glorious red Christmas colours, and the sky was a dazzling blue, I could hardly enjoy them in the eternity she was out of my sight. I was very relieved when she came back, probably only 20 minutes later! She had obviously enjoyed herself. Another connecting beam in the Bridge of Trust had been built.

Something that had come to me while working with one young man was the idea that we can hold two different perspectives in our heads about something at the same time. This young man believed that most people hated him and wanted him dead because he had such an important role to play in with world,

'A bit like Jesus', he said.

He thought there was a plot to murder him, and at times he would become verbally aggressive as a result of this fear, even though he tried his best to be more 'like Jesus'. There was very little, if any, eye contact, but he was prepared to sit with me in the interview room if I brought us both a cup of tea or coffee.

On a piece of paper, I drew him a line-drawing of a stick person with two overlapping elliptical shapes over its head, a bit like a Venn diagram. He was prepared to look at this picture rather than looking at me. I had explained that sometimes our upsetting beliefs can seem absolutely true in some circumstances, but if we can challenge them and find out what's really going on, actually that can help us feel better. As a child, I had been febrile and delirious, and I still remembered the vivid visions of animals I had seen in my room. I shared this memory with him. It turned out that he had a similar experience, as many children do. I used this as an example of how our mind and brain can play tricks on us, with two different versions of reality. I showed him, using my little diagram, how one set of beliefs could be very real on the one hand (as represented by one ellipse), but viewed from another perspective (the other ellipse), things can look different. I explained that psychosis is a bit like that and that the illness called 'schizophrenia' can play similar tricks, making us believe things that aren't always true. He expressed relief at the possibility that his belief that people wanted him dead was not true, but it was hard for him to hold on to this new perspective.

At the same time, it became clear to him during our low-key conversations over cups of tea or coffee that maybe he would miss the feeling of being so special, if he no longer held the belief that people wanted him dead.

'But I know I have something special to do. God has a plan for my life', he said.

'Yes', I agreed. 'Let's see if together we can find out what that is!'

Sometimes he would misinterpret my actions or the tone of my voice while we were chatting in this way, believing that I was being hostile and rejecting. At these times, he would become verbally aggressive and refuse to see me. My willingness to continue to approach him with the offer of a cup of tea gradually overcame his doubts about my trustworthiness. Sitting alongside each other, we could gently explore his feelings. Gradually he became able to identify his fear of social situations and a belief that he would be deliberately humiliated. He recalled having been bullied as a child. He talked about his loneliness and need for social contact. He had been isolated in his starkly barren hospital room for almost two years since his admission.

Within the context of many seemingly ordinary social conversations, we explored his upsetting beliefs about people wanting him dead, often looking at the little diagram that I would draw on a serviette to remind him of how we can hold different views of the same thing at the same time. After many meetings on the ward, we ventured out to a local café. The Bridge of Trust stretched with us, allowing more and more confidence to build on both sides. He began to pay more attention to his appearance, began to take showers. He put a picture on his wall – something he had found in a magazine with clouds and a rainbow. Staff noticed he was making more eye contact and responded by greeting him with a wave and a smile when they saw him. He smiled and laughed more. He agreed for the hospital chaplain to visit him and eventually began to attend church services.

Eventually, after 203 meetings, and I don't know how many cups of tea or coffee, he took up a job in the local gardens and began to learn horticulture. He had always enjoyed growing seedlings when he was younger.

'Maybe I'm meant to be a gardener', he said.

'Yes!' I said, with a little smile.

I wondered whether he was aware of the scripture that refers to Jesus as the gardener. Maybe he was beginning to find a plan for his life. At times, his fears and hostility would resurface under certain stressful situations, but by now he knew how to keep himself and others safe by taking himself off to his room to listen to Christian music or write in his journal.

Looking back, I can see that the number of sessions I spent with the nine people over the years of my research was only possible because of the nature of my role at the time. When I spoke about my work, other psychiatrists used to say that hundreds of sessions were unachievable for them. At the time, this didn't seem important, as what I was doing seemed to be changing people's lives. To the reader, too, it may seem that 203 or 173 meetings would be impossible in usual clinical settings. However, if every interaction (even very brief ones) from every person working in mental health were therapeutically attuned in these ways, who knows what the outcomes could be? This was the direction I hoped might be possible for mental health services. Over the intervening decades since then, I have developed ways of achieving these sorts of changes in fewer hours and with additive contributions from all the people involved in each person's care, not just a specific therapist. As the Buchanan Rehabilitation Centre (BRC) evolved, all staff began working along similar lines. I am continuing to develop resources to support conversations to be as useful as they can be.

Where I am up to at the time of writing this book is 'The Gift Box', a repository for all I have learned, which I hope will soon become available to support wellbeing on a global scale.

In my research, I used my little Venn diagram in an attempt to give a helpful alternative explanation to each person about the possible nature of their experiences. I combined the idea of building the Bridge of Trust with this diagram, explaining that I wanted to cross over this Bridge of Trust, to see things as clearly as possible from their perspective. Then I might be able to show them how I saw things from my perspective, as we built this bridge.

For example, one man spent many hours talking of his memories of complex and detailed childhood exploits involving 'gazillions of dollars', and hidden treasures as well as extreme dangers. I could never get a clear picture of what he had actually endured, but I supposed whatever it was must have been unbearable for him, and he had done his best to make it into a meaningful story for himself. I would always try to validate and normalise what I intuited he must have felt, given the experiences he told me about.

For example, I would say things like, 'It sounds as if you had to be very brave to get through all that'. He would acknowledge that this was true, with a satisfied look of recognition. I explained that the descriptions seemed a bit dream-like, and that psychosis is like a waking dream. I asked him if he noticed that now he was on clozapine (a medication that was only used as a last resort because of potentially fatal side effects), he no longer found himself experiencing the sort of unusual adventures he recalled from his childhood. He acknowledged that the clozapine was helping him feel more relaxed and more able to focus in the here and now. After retelling me his version of his life story many times, with me listening actively and patiently, he gradually became less preoccupied with these 'memories' and more able to focus on meaningful activity, eventually getting a paid job in a local agency for supported employment, and moving out of the hospital into supported accommodation.

I would draw my spiral diagram to explain the concept of 're-covery', talking with each person about how patterns that tend to repeat themselves can change in positive ways given the right support. An example of this was when I assisted people who had a pattern of being unsociable or hostile towards others. I guided them in learning basic talking and listening skills with appropriate use of facial expression. As they used these skills, for example, making eye contact and smiling more, other people responded more warmly towards them, and they experienced improvements in relationships. Consequently, their confidence and self-esteem improved. It often turned out that these people had been bullied. They were now learning to re-cover the old ground of what used to be upsetting contact with others, in new and encouraging ways.

One man believed he was suffering from life-threatening infectious diseases which made him febrile. As a result, he isolated himself and refused to engage in activities. Eventually, because he had gradually learned to trust me by experiencing the quality of our 'being with' one another, he was willing to check his temperature with a thermometer each time he felt hot, thus demonstrating to himself that his assumption of fever and illness was unfounded. He began to notice that when he felt hot, he had usually experienced a situation that was stressful, such as having to get to an appointment on time when he had other important things to do as well. I normalised and validated his response, acknowledging repeatedly that it was not surprising that he felt a bit 'hot and bothered' when things like that happened in life, and I often felt like that too. He became willing to consider that other aspects of his upsetting beliefs might also have other explanations, and eventually became less anxious and generally more trusting.

In the context of 'being with' people, I helped them to identify and manage other upsetting emotional states. One woman told me she was having panic attacks when any demand was made on her to perform tasks, such as making dinner. What she meant by 'panic attacks' was a feeling of needing to get away from the upsetting situation. She would retire to her bedroom complaining of headaches and subsequently hear indistinct voices. Gradually she became more able to notice what she was feeling and name it as 'fear and anxiety'. She self-soothed by practising relaxation techniques that I taught her, having learned my own ways of calming myself, such as tummy breathing. She would tell herself that with help she could learn to do many things. Eventually, she mastered many everyday tasks that previously she had avoided. This particular young woman never opened up about her early life experiences or what had happened to her, and I respected that the time was not right for her to do that.

Another 'modality', based on what I had learned in my own journey, was to explore with each person in the research group, the importance that they placed on spiritual and religious issues. Often people would tell me long and interesting stories of their spiritual and religious development from early childhood and what that meant to them now.

After 21 months, and hundreds of sessions spent with each person, all nine participants in my research had improved so much that they were able to leave hospital. They did strikingly better than a matched comparison group of 12 other people without my intervention. Discovering that their assessment results were also *statistically* better than the control group was like a miracle. All my painstaking efforts to produce a scientifically rigorous study had paid off. Despite all the doubts about my own ability, it really did seem as if God was going with me and giving me success in my work after all. Although it was to take several more years, I was able to get the research written up and eventually published (Randal et al., 2003).

19

SOMETHING WRONG ON THE INSIDE

The Paradox

In which Patte excels in being a 'good patient' with very mixed results.

Given the positive outcomes of my research, it felt a bit of a mystery to me that life continued to feel such an uphill struggle. Up until my decision to take regular risperidone, which happened to coincide with the start of the research, I had always felt joy in the work I was doing. Following my passion – my dream – of making a contribution to psychiatry was what gave my life meaning, but this felt almost the opposite. Cam was always supportive and kind to me, encouraging me to take one step at a time. I would not have got through it without him.

But feeling so flat most of the time did not have the flavour of a life worth living, even though, on the outside, I was 'successful'. It was a paradox. The outward success did not match my internal experience. I hadn't even told my psychiatrist what was happening, because I believed it was my own fault for taking on such a huge project. I was now completing this herculean task, but I felt that I'd lost the sense of pathway, as if I'd been defeated in the spiritual battle. I kept thinking that this research was my attempt to fulfil my own destiny in my own strength, and I had a horrible feeling that it had backfired on me. I could hardly believe it would really amount to anything.

Looking back as I write this in 2020, I wonder whether this loss of a positive sense of meaning might have been due to an unrecognised side effect of the risperidone? What I now suspect is that this tiny white tablet was draining my sense of joy and causing an overall feeling of reduced meaning and purpose in my life.

One known effect of 'antipsychotic' medications like risperidone is that they block dopamine, a neurotransmitter in the brain. According to one theory, a central role of the naturally occurring dopamine in the brain is to mediate the 'salience' of environmental events and representations (Kapur, 2003). In other words, it might be said that dopamine is involved in creating the lived experience of meaning-making. In my extreme states, everything felt more

DOI: 10.4324/9781003153788-28

meaningful. Colours were brighter; the juxtaposition of events seemed more and more 'synchronous', as if everything had become much more salient, and hidden meaning became apparent.

For example, I remember once crossing the road and a traffic light turned red. That meant much more to me than simply a sign to stop walking. It meant I had to stop doing some activity in my life. In a flash, I concluded that I was to end a friendship with a particular person. I was jumping to the wrong conclusion about the meaning of the red stop light. Maybe during that extreme state, I had more dopamine than usual circulating around my brain, rather like at times when we are stressed or excited, we have more adrenaline in our bodies. We all know what an adrenaline rush feels like.

It may be that dopamine-blocking drugs such as risperidone actually block that meaning-making pathway and can thereby block what Kapur calls 'aberrant salience'. What this phrase refers to is the attribution of idiosyncratic (or 'off track') meaning. In the example about the traffic lights, dopamine blockade would result in reducing the likelihood of jumping to the wrong conclusion about what it meant when the traffic light turned red.

If that is the case, then maybe because I have an extremely sensitive nervous system, the risperidone also blocked *everyday/on track* salience (as well as blocking *aberrant/off track* salience). I now suspect that what made it so hard for me when I was doing the research was that this effect also led to *everything* feeling less meaningful and much harder to manage on a day-to-day basis. The feeling of being on track, that encouraging sense of pathway that I relied on to guide me, seemed to have evaporated. That is how it felt. It was a bit like having the volume, brightness, and colour of my life turned right down. However, at the time, the possibility had not occurred to me that the tiny dose of risperidone might be implicated.

When I did finally go to see my psychiatrist, she said she had not realised how bad I was feeling. I could suddenly see that any psychiatrist would understand that what was happening to me was a depressive swing. Until that time, it had not crossed my mind that this was the explanation for how hard it all felt. I remember talking about myself with my psychiatrist as a colleague would about a patient. Like Josephine, it was as if my doctor-self suddenly took over and joined with my psychiatrist in the role of treating me as a patient. Together we came to the conclusion that, looking back over the years and counting the number of episodes, as well as noticing the pattern of my mood with times of euphoria, times of terror, and times of anguish, it would fit with a diagnosis of Bipolar Disorder. This took into account the fact that my psychiatrist had consulted Tony Ryle who had said that he thought my first episode back in 1976 had been 'hypomania'.

In joining with my psychiatrist as a fellow doctor, and treating myself from that perspective, I put aside my notions of re-framing my own experience of psychosis as a mystical, spiritual emergency. I stopped believing that what I had experienced in my extreme states made sense in terms of what had happened to me. I disregarded the cry of my heart in just the same way that I had earlier felt that psychiatry had disregarded me. All I wanted was to feel better. It was an opportunity to begin to see eye-to-eye with Cam. We were both doctors. We could both see things from a medical perspective. Cam was well able and willing to support me in a shared perspective of me having a diagnosis of Bipolar Disorder.

Given the extremity of my suffering over the previous two years, my psychiatrist suggested that it was time for me to take antidepressant medication in addition to the risperidone. Unfortunately, the first one we tried, paroxetine, caused the worst experience I've ever endured, making me feel as if I was literally jumping out of my skin. I could not keep still; it was as if my body were flying apart at the seams. Going through this nightmarish time seemed to make everything else a million times worse, especially as I initially thought it was part of the 'illness', rather than a side effect of the treatment! Eventually, we found a combination of medication that helped me feel calmer and more settled, and to sleep well. I was so relieved. Although in many ways my inner world felt so limited and uninspiring, I was more relaxed. I could get on with my life adequately, even though the passion and sparkle had gone.

Important things were happening in my marriage around this time, too. Cam and I had bought a holiday home overlooking a magnificent view of the sea with green hills in the near distance, a short walk from a secluded beach. It was a dream place and we began to spend weekends there with the children. I believed that this peaceful refuge would become somewhere I would eventually be able to share my faith journey with Cam, and that we would form a deeper understanding of one another.

However, Cam confided in me that he had loving feelings for one of the women with whom he worked. Despite our love for one another, I had always on some level felt insecure in my marriage and this overt admission was very unnerving. Somehow, however, I managed to allow him to talk with me about this without freaking out. I validated him. It touched me that Cam would trust me enough to share his experience with me, but it left me feeling much more insecure than before. This woman was married at the time and both she and her husband had a Christian faith. They had reached out to me as a fellow 'follower of Jesus'. On the surface, I felt encouraged by the idea that they might share their faith with Cam. Underneath that superficial acceptance, however, I felt afraid. I could not bear the thought of losing my darling husband. From around that time I would occasionally hear an inner 'voice' telling me: *Cam will have an affair*.

Once I was on the combination of risperidone and antidepressants, I needed Cam more than ever. I was in a diminished and sometimes anxious state and he continued as ever to be supportive and loving towards me. I suspect that it was easier for him to know that I was safely medicated than to live with the fear that I might have a relapse. The cost for me was enormous in terms of my ability to function fully and creatively. However, as the years unfolded with no further episodes of psychosis or extreme states, we both began to accept the status quo. We both came to believe that indeed I had Bipolar Disorder and being on medication for the rest of my life was not a high price to pay for my 'sanity'. Despite my underlying insecurities, our Bridge of Trust appeared to be solid and durable.

20

FINDING MY VOICE ... AND LOSING IT AGAIN

In which Patte learns from others with lived experience, begins to speak out about her own recovery from psychosis and has a rude awakening.

Kay Redfield Jamison is an international authority on 'manic-depressive illness' (or Bipolar Disorder). In 1995, at the height of her career, she published a memoir of her own struggle with extreme mood states. In her book, *An Unquiet Mind* (Jamison, 1996), she revealed her vulnerability in a moving way. Because I was fascinated by her revelations about herself, I did a presentation on her book in a journal club. I was surprised to find myself feeling uncomfortable about not acknowledging that I too had experienced extreme states. It was a scary thing to do.

I wondered if, by telling my story, I could get people to think differently about psychosis and recovery. Other people with experience of mental illness were starting to speak out about it too. On the world stage, what became known as the 'Recovery Movement' (Davidson, 2016) was beginning to emerge. Speaking out for those who had no voice was part of it; people who, like me, had been rejected or discriminated against because of the extreme states we had endured.

I wanted to show people that doctors are just like everyone else on some human level, and that finding our professional place is possible even after such apparently catastrophic events. Potentially we can be a conduit for healing when we are prepared to *collaborate with* our therapeutic partners, rather than *doing things to* them in the name of *treatment*. It felt purposeful and meaningful to begin speaking out.

It seemed particularly important to demonstrate that extreme states can be triggered by situations that do not make sense or are somehow linked with re-covering repeated patterns of broken trust. And that trust can be rebuilt, and healing can happen. Explaining the impact of what happened to me as a psychiatry registrar was such a clear example. On the one hand, I had been acknowledged for my ideas, theoretical frameworks and practices, and on

 DOI: 10.4324/9781003153788-29

the other hand I had been rejected because my ideas differed from my senior colleagues'. I wanted to show how the extreme state of psychosis followed this paradoxical experience. Blame was not on my mind. The whole sequence had simply reflected the state of the art back then.

My opportunity arose in 1998 when I heard about the Building Bridges conference that was due to take place in Hobart, Tasmania. It would not have felt safe for me just to tell my story, because I knew there was a risk that I might be seen as lacking credibility if I simply presented what had happened to me. Kay Redfield Jamison was protected by her professional status. People were prepared to listen to her because they respected her. So, I decided to give two papers. One was an academic presentation. It was about the positive outcomes of my therapeutic work and the intervention research that I had begun. The other was my personal story, titled *Building Bridges, or Why I No Longer Have to Walk on Water*. Debbie attended the conference with me; I could not have done it without her.

I began by saying: 'Today I want to talk about how I learned and am still learning to build bridges. I want to take the risk of building a bridge from where I am to where you are. A Bridge of Trust'.

I talked about my impression that there were a number of bridge-builders who were making it possible for Mental Health Services to offer better, more hopeful options for people with serious mental illness. I acknowledged that some, including me, have our own personal experiences of survival while also working as clinicians and researchers. I wondered whether we might have some special bridge-building skills that we had learned along the way, and that we could use to teach others.

I still feel proud of what I said.

> A bridge is necessary when there is a gap between one place and another. In Western culture there has been such a gap between 'the mentally ill' and everyone else. Psychotic illness, particularly, has seemed to create a sense of a gap between the reality of the sufferer and the reality of the world. That gap has been the source of much suffering for those people with mental illness, their families and society at large. It is a gap that has been filled with lack of trust; fear and anger; confusion and chaos. Although mental health professionals have done their best to span that gap with various understandings based on the bio-psycho-social model, we have been left with the stigma and discrimination which seems to make the suffering of mental illness so much worse.

Then I told the story of how what happened to me in psychiatry had almost destroyed me, and how my new-found faith was strengthening me. As the conference progressed, a lot of positive feedback reached me. I returned from Tasmania feeling both my talks were a success. I had broken a taboo, rebelling against the culture of medicine that had us hiding our vulnerability. We had been taught to act as if we were super-people who did not get sick, specially not mentally ill and definitely not psychotic. Looking back, I think I was a bit of an unseen pioneer in the vanguard of this growing Recovery Movement.

As my research time was drawing to a close in 1999, Buchanan Clinic hosted a training visit from Laurie Curtis, an American international leader of the fledgling Recovery Movement. I enjoyed the course immensely and resonated with what she taught. Most of her material felt uncannily familiar to me because of my own lived experience. At the end of the course, she detailed a dazzling list of academic and clinical achievements belonging to person A on one whiteboard, and an equally dazzling list of hospital admissions, medications, and diagnoses belonging to person B on another whiteboard. We were given some minutes to consider how we might respond to each of these two people. Laurie then quietly told us that both lists were descriptions of her own life experiences. I was struck by her courage and felt validated in the choice I had made to speak out.

Laurie put forward a list of recovery principles, the most important of which was 'hope'. We were challenged with the task of figuring out how to instil hope into the lives of the people we serve. She also brought us Patricia Deegan's ideas about how psychiatry could be spirit-breaking; and that crises are opportunities for change. Patricia Deegan had been given a diagnosis of 'schizophrenia' as a young woman and spent many years in a back ward in an American asylum. Her writing about what she endured is poignant. She described sitting in a chair, smoking incessantly. For her, 'giving up' was a way of surviving. If she had no hope, she could not be disappointed any more. This was a powerful, lingering image. Eventually, a flame of hope was mysteriously rekindled for her. She was able to make a personal recovery and trained to be a clinical psychologist (Deegan, 1996).

Through her writing I recognised the meaning of a lot of the behaviour I'd witnessed in the people I served – the loss of motivation, and diminished emotional and interpersonal responsiveness that psychiatrists call 'negative symptoms'. In my clinical practice and my research, I found ways of supporting people as I held the hope for them. Being with people in an accepting, validating way helped them realise that they do matter. Rather than being spirit-breaking, it helped them to hope again. The Recovery Movement had its emphasis on empowerment, self-responsibility, self-advocacy, education, support and finding purpose and meaning – all validating my own understanding of the spiral of 're-covery' that I had been developing since the late-eighties. This was another affirmation that I was on the right track.

While I was doing my research, Buchanan Clinic transformed from a custodial care unit into a new service which embraced the recovery approach. For several years, I took part in delivering various recovery training workshops to the staff, based on Laurie Curtis and Patricia Deegan's teachings. Staff – who had until then walked around with huge heavy metal keys that kept people locked within rooms and wards – learned new ways of being with those people to maintain safety more effectively and humanely. At this stage I did not incorporate my own 're-covery' concept into my teaching.

In 1999, a version of my personal story was published as one of 22 narratives in the New Zealand book, *A Gift of Stories*, compiled by Dr Julie Leibrich (Leibrich, 1999). As the first Mental Health Commissioner with lived experience herself, Julie has been an important contributor to the Recovery Movement. She has become a personal friend, and I know that *A Gift of Stories* has been a hugely positive influence in many ways – locally and globally. Wendy Harrex of Otago University Press was the publisher, along with the Mental Health Commission. Coincidentally, it had been Wendy, working for a different publishing company back in 1990, who had read my original autobiographical novel. When I realised that Wendy was the publisher of *A Gift of Stories*, it felt to me as if a power beyond me was conspiring to get my story out into the world.

At the time my story was published in Julie's book, I was feeling quite despondent, believing that I had a 'mental illness' and would need to be on medication for the rest of my life. I later came to wonder whether much of my reduced capacity had actually been *caused* by the medication I was taking. I had always suffered such anxiety in my role as a doctor over the possibility that my actions could cause harm. When, some years after it was published, I was given a copy of the book by a drug rep from the company that made risperidone, it crossed my mind all too uncomfortably that I, as a contributor to the book, had indirectly supported the drug company's marketing efforts. The issue of medication is not emphasised in the book and, in my story, I didn't specifically name risperidone as the medication I was taking. Nevertheless, one of the messages *I* gave was that medication was a lifelong necessity for people who had endured extreme states as I had. In saying this, I am running ahead of myself, but it is *this* message that I now regret. Perhaps part of the motivation to publish this book is connected with my desire to tell the whole story; to be re-covering the same ground in a new way. As Wendy Harrex had said, when she read my autobiographical novel written all those years before I was on regular medication: 'It's a story that needs to be told'.

In 2002, I featured with three other women in a New Zealand television documentary titled 'Four Women', as part of the *Inside Out series (Point of View Productions, 2002)*. This episode took the hopeful perspective that recovery and a life worth living are possible for people diagnosed with so-called schizophrenia and Bipolar Disorder. There was a clip in the movie of me wearing my smartest clothes and checking blood forms in the clinic, as once I had completed my research, this had become part of my medical role. I was grateful to have another opportunity to help reduce stigma and discrimination, to be able to demonstrate that someone diagnosed with a 'mental illness' could work as a doctor. But I was bewildered when I noticed, watching the broadcast, that every time I attempted to talk, there was tension and spasm in my vocal cords. I did not know what caused this.

Around the time that *A Gift of Stories* was published, I began to attend the Hearing Voices groups that were being facilitated in Auckland District Health Board by Miriam Loretto and Debra Lampshire. I was there to learn this exciting and creative approach to addressing upsetting voices, as part of my recovery training. Debra is inspiring in so many ways. She has lived experience of voice-hearing and earlier in her life was diagnosed as having 'schizophrenia'. She has become a major leader in the global Hearing Voices movement, heralding the initiation of an international organisation that recognises voice-hearing as a valid and universal human experience. Rather like Patricia Deegan, Debra has a remarkable story of recovery from extreme states in which she was paralysed by voices and trapped in the back wards of a New Zealand psychiatric hospital. From what I recall of Debra's story, some of the voices would tell her she was to be a world leader. Her teaching, her charismatic personality and her hilarious storytelling have indeed made her a much-loved world leader in her field. She now teaches at the University of Auckland, telling her story publicly in many settings including a TED talk. Although I am not a voice-hearer myself, I can honestly say that I learned more from Debra than from any of my 'psychiatry training' – most of which I needed to unlearn to become effective in the endeavour of supporting recovery. Debra taught me about using my own lived experience as a tool, although it was to be some time before I incorporated that into my clinical practice.

When I sat in on the Hearing Voices groups that Debra co-facilitated with Miriam, a nurse, they were using a diagram depicting what is known as the five-part model. I later learned that this was developed by Christine Padesky (Greenberger & Padesky, 1995). They used this diagram to demonstrate how to identify the elements of stressful situations that can lead to upsetting voices. This was a pivotal learning experience for me, both personally and in my clinical and educator role.

For example (see Figure 20.1), if someone is in the situation of 'being stood up on a date', they might experience body sensations such as 'feeling nausea'. They might identify emotional feelings such as 'fear and anxiety' and thoughts like, 'I'll never get a girlfriend. I'll be lonely all my life'. A voice might follow, saying, 'You make me sick. Loser!' Then actions such as 'withdrawing and refusing to go out' might ensue, with their own mix of both helpful and unhelpful consequences. The process of identifying all the individual pieces of what might be an overwhelming experience can give the person a chance to process them on a manageable level. This has the potential to interrupt a vicious cycle where body sensations, thoughts, feelings, and actions feed each other, and allows the person to address each piece one by one.

Debra talked about voice-hearing as 'clunky communication' – as if from a friend who wanted to protect the person from something unpleasant but

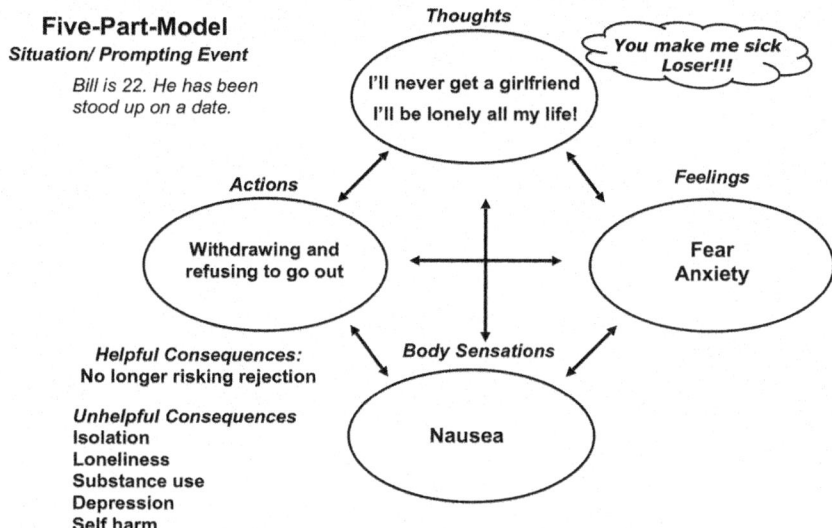

Figure 20.1 Five-part model showing 'clunky communication'.

did so in a clunky and often counterproductive way. In this case, the voice saying, 'You make me sick. Loser!' might be a well-meaning attempt to keep the voice-hearer from venturing out and potentially being rejected again. Unfortunately, the consequences might be far worse, such as increasing isolation, loneliness, substance use, depression, and self-harm.

Observing Miriam and Debra workshopping in their teaching roles was yet another *aha* experience for me. I was beginning to understand more about how our minds work, and the way the emotional impact of our interpretation of situations affects our actions. I was beginning to piece together how things could build up into extreme states, way beyond what people consider 'normal'. And yet all this made complete sense. It seemed as if it might happen to anyone under extreme enough circumstances. It gave us a meaningful pathway to normalise and validate voice-hearing. And I could see that the same would be true for extreme beliefs, such as I had experienced when I was psychotic.

Some of what I learned from Debra was helpful to me in a personal way. Because I had thought I had to be superhuman and cope with everything perfectly, I hadn't allowed myself to acknowledge when terrifying situations were causing me stress. An example of this is when I was confronted by the two professors telling me I was not going to be reappointed as a registrar. Using the five-part model can help make more sense of the sequence of events leading to the extreme-state experience that followed this meeting (see Figure 20.2).

After I had been told I was too open and honest and had too much integrity to be a psychiatrist in Auckland ('*the situation', or 'prompting event'*), the

151

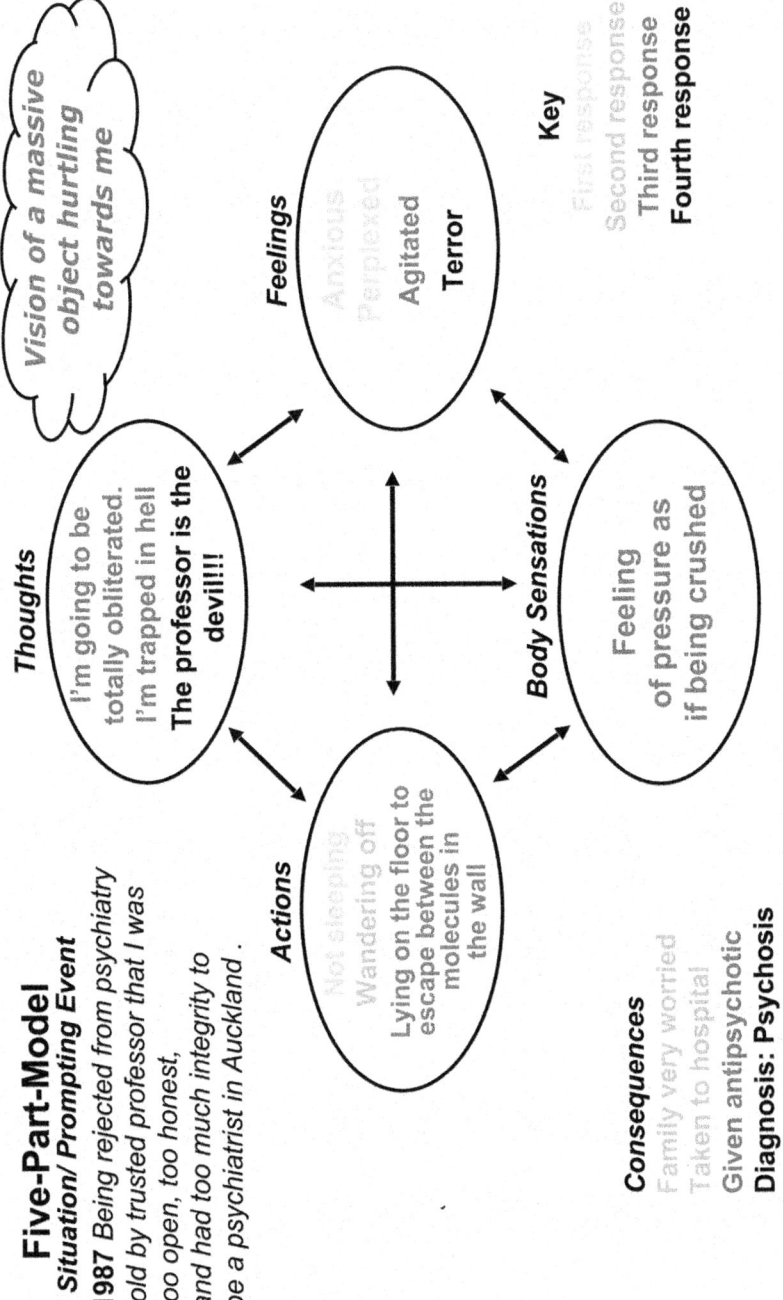

Five-Part-Model
Situation/ Prompting Event
1987 *Being rejected from psychiatry told by trusted professor that I was too open, too honest, and had too much integrity to be a psychiatrist in Auckland .*

Thoughts

I'm going to be totally obliterated.
I'm trapped in hell
The professor is the devil!!!

Feelings

Anxious
Perplexed
Agitated
Terror

Key
First response
Second response
Third response
Fourth response

Body Sensations

Feeling
of pressure as
if being crushed

Actions

Not sleeping
Wandering off
Lying on the floor to escape between the molecules in the wall

Consequences
Family very worried
Taken to hospital
Given antipsychotic
Diagnosis: Psychosis

Figure 20.2 Five-part model showing sequence leading to extreme state.

152

stress of it all (*'body sensations'* and *'feelings'*) had the effect that I didn't sleep for three nights (*'actions'*). I experienced the impending sense or vision of being crushed and obliterated by a gigantic moon-sized ball bearing racing towards me (*'thoughts'*). When I am stressed, a common body sensation is a sense of crushing pressure in my chest. Maybe this links back to my childhood strategy of holding my breath so as not to cry. Using the five-part model has helped me figure out that the feeling of crushing pressure in my chest was my body telling me that I was feeling anxious, or pressured, or even crushed. In this particular situation, I was indeed metaphorically being crushed by the shock of being thrown out of psychiatry by the same trusted person who had previously validated me so positively. On the level of what was happening physiologically, the jigsaw puzzle meaning of the symbolism falls into place.

To this day, if I notice that uncomfortable feeling in my chest, it is often the earliest warning of something stressful. Often I have not even noticed the stressor. So when I'm aware of this physical feeling, I need to stop and reflect. Usually it will be something that has triggered me. For example, being under pressure; too many things changing at once; or being in a conflict that feels too hard to resolve. If I manage to notice this pattern, I can take special care of myself and not get overwhelmed. It really helps.

Another major influence which helped transform my clinical and personal practice, was dialectical behaviour therapy (DBT), one of the leading therapies for people with repeated suicidal and self-harm behaviour. Many years after this approach had received global recognition, Marsha Linehan disclosed that her own recovery journey underpinned the therapy she created. Buddhist ideas and practices were an important part of this. Much like Laurie Curtis, Patricia Deegan, and Debra Lampshire, her personal experience of extreme states enabled her to make a major transformational impact on the world. I feel fortunate to have had so many opportunities for expert training. I never met Marsha herself, but in 2000 I was able to engage in a training in DBT with her team.

One piece of the DBT approach, which came easily and intuitively to me, was the warm and generous building of a therapeutic relationship. I became much more consciously competent at the skill of validation. This meant radical acceptance of the person, their feelings, and experiences. I found the clear structure of the approach helped contain my anxiety as a clinician when confronted by serious suicidal behaviour. I didn't have to figure it out each time someone attempted suicide, or was making plans to self-harm. The steps we needed to take in each therapy session were laid out for both me and the person with whom I was engaging. We both knew the rules and had agreed to follow them at the outset. Learning how to apply these rules was rather like being given a map when you are lost. Suddenly you can find your way out of an otherwise hopeless situation. This was yet another *aha* experience for me.

I also attended a workshop led by Charles Rapp. His focus on strengths further helped me unlearn the pathologising orientation of my psychiatry training. In retrospect, this was an enriching period of my professional life. I was incorporating everything I was learning into my own clinical practice. Despite this though, I was still struggling with a reduced sense of meaning. Then something strange happened.

By 2001, I was beginning to notice that, physically, it required increasingly more effort to speak. My work was becoming more difficult because of this. By this time, I had completed my research and was employed in my area of expertise as a non-specialist hospital psychiatrist for people who had long-term and intractable issues. My speech problem continued to worsen to the point where I could hardly make myself heard, especially when I spoke on the phone, or when there was noise in the room. In social settings such as cafes, conversation became increasingly impossible. I would need to choose every word carefully because of the immense physical effort. It was frustrating and exhausting.

Eventually this was diagnosed as a condition known as 'spasmodic dys-phonia', which simply means that the muscles that generate the voice go into spasm. The cause is generally unknown. However, I realised in collaboration with a neurologist and an Ear, Nose, and Throat specialist that, in my case, this was an exceedingly rare form of drug side effect known as a 'tardive dys-tonia', a form of brain damage affecting the basal ganglia. The word 'tardive' means slow onset, and 'dystonia' means involuntary muscle contractions.

In my case, this side effect affecting my voice was caused by taking the tiny dose of risperidone (0.5 mg), possibly in combination with the antidepressants (citalopram and nortriptyline). My psychiatrist and I co-authored a letter about it that was later published in a psychiatry journal. This condition was deemed a medical mishap and I was eventually awarded compensation. I had to stop work on medical grounds because the effort of talking made my work impossible. To lose this vital ability of speech was catastrophic – physically, professionally, and relationally. And yet so much of value eventually came out of it.

I had by now experienced two rare, and very serious, toxic side effects of small doses of frequently prescribed 'antipsychotics'. In retrospect I can see that there may have been a third hidden side effect impacting my capacity for meaning-making. These personal experiences reinforced my already strong caution about prescribing the medications we routinely use in psychiatry. It was a lesson that was to change my life and my clinical practice irreversibly. Having found my place as a clinician, therapist, published researcher, and as a person who would speak out for those who had no voice, I had literally lost mine. And not only had I lost the voice that I had so recently metaphor-ically found, but also, for the second time in my career in psychiatry, I was re-covering the unwanted experience of losing my place once again. What sense could I make of all this?

21

SIDE EFFECTS, SPIRITUALITY, AND FINDING MY NICHE

In which one door closes and others open and Patte finds a new way forward

To my surprise, it was a relief to stop work. Firstly, because I could avoid the physical effort of talking to people. Secondly, working as a non-specialist psychiatrist, I'd been routinely required to prescribe 'antipsychotic' medications. Over the years, since qualifying as a doctor, I had endured many sleepless nights worrying 'what if'. Everything I prescribed inevitably had side effects. The responsibility weighed heavily on me. I never wanted to harm people. In psychiatry, we believed better medications with fewer side effects were becoming available. Also, we were using lower doses, and monitoring to avoid potentially lethal effects from drugs such as clozapine. Back then, we didn't know about the extreme problems that were to emerge with the metabolic syndrome that now plagues the use of the newer medications (Mazereel, Detraux, Vancampfort, van Winkel, & De Hert, 2020). I had obediently taken the risperidone tablets, believing the drug company's marketing ploy about its safety profile, which turned out to be untrue. While I was taking it, I didn't have a psychotic episode for six years. I would have carried on taking them forever if this voice problem hadn't happened. Living through yet another such debilitating side effect myself, I found it profoundly disturbing to be exposing other people to these risks. In a way, I was glad it was happening to me rather than one of the people for whom I had prescribed this medication.

Once I realised the damage the pills had done to me, I very cautiously began to reduce the already tiny doses, gradually weaning myself off them with my psychiatrist's approval. My role model was a close friend (also a doctor) who herself had courageously taken this road less travelled. I continued for a while longer with the antidepressant (citalopram). Despite my misgivings about taking the risperidone, I was also somewhat fearful of the consequences of coming off all medication. Cam was also concerned about what might happen. Neither of us wanted a recurrence of the psychosis, and usually people with a diagnosis of Bipolar Disorder stay on mood stabilising medication for life.

DOI: 10.4324/9781003153788-30

My voice did not improve at all once I stopped taking the risperidone. Unfortunately, this type of side effect is usually chronic and difficult to treat. Some of my psychiatrist colleagues and friends suggested alternative medications, which might have helped rectify my voice problem as well as protecting me from further episodes of psychosis. One such suggestion was to take clozapine, which has so many life-threatening and quality-of-life threatening side effects, and it is only used if other treatments fail. Heaven knows what might have happened to me if I had taken that!

What was I going to do now that my oral communication was so limited? I decided to get another puppy. We already had our beautiful dog, Buffy, the sleek and cheeky English Pointer. I had often thought she would be better off with a companion. Now I had the free time to enjoy the challenge and fun of training two dogs. We chose Ella, a chocolate and cream German Shorthaired Pointer. These two furry friends were a great distraction for me, although I never managed to get them to be totally obedient, as I could not use my voice to train them. Nevertheless, they were great 'sick-leave' companions, and we all loved them. Our daily walks helped to keep us all fit and they made me laugh with their merry antics.

I also used my time to focus on writing up my research. I'd submitted a version to the Schizophrenia Bulletin, but it had been turned down. It was Josephine who persuaded me to get my research findings into the public domain. Given the space for reflection, I was able to clarify the details of my knowledge and learning that had informed my approach with each individual. All the training I had done in the interim, together with reading about the emerging work of other researchers in this field, helped me to conceptualise what I had intuitively known was needed. Eventually, in 2003, my research was published in the Australian and New Zealand Journal of Psychiatry. It seemed a bit of a miracle.

The other small miracle during my 'time off' was that I was awarded a grant by the Mental Health Commission to write a paper on spirituality and mental health. I had interpreted my first extreme state as a 'mystical experience'. After the second episode in 1986, I read a book called Spiritual Emergency (Groff & Groff, 1989), and this term became part of my vocabulary because it captured the essence of what I felt had happened to me. Writing the paper for the commission gave me the opportunity to revisit the ideas that I had put aside when I took on the diagnosis of Bipolar Disorder and capitulated to the 'medical model'. I was able to get in touch with many of the people globally who had published their thoughts about this concept. I argued that the whole spectrum of extreme states, from brief psychotic episodes to so-called schizophrenia, schizoaffective disorder, and Bipolar Disorder, could be addressed as spiritual (or meaning-making) emergencies. In my view, this approach has the potential to support better mental health and well-being. My premise was that the extreme-state crisis could be an opportunity for greater self-awareness and transformation, given the right input.

The responses I received, including letters and emails from all over the world, were very encouraging. Many people took the trouble to critique my writing and add their perspective. It was exhilarating to belong to an international group who were all taking seriously the potential for extreme states to be healing experiences. With some tentativeness, we all saw the need for these ideas to be brought into the arena of ordinary mental health care so as to inform better practice.

Feeling personally happy with the finished product, I submitted the paper. Two senior psychiatrists reviewed it. I was shocked and yes – angered – to hear that they refused to allow it to be published. I was re-covering the same old ground of invalidation and rejection of my ideas and theoretical frameworks. Jim Wright encouraged me to get the paper published anyway, but I had lost my nerve. Privately, I decided to incorporate the concepts into my own understanding. I was so aware of the importance of my own spiritual emergence and how strengthening that was proving to be after so many devastating emergencies (spiritual and otherwise) in my life. I'm happy to say that in 2005, a revised version of that paper, co-authored with Dr Nick Argyle, was published on the British Royal College of Psychiatry Special Interest Group website (Randal & Argyle, 2005).

With Debbie's support, in late 2002, I began to take very gradual steps to re-establish myself in a new role at the hospital. As a result of my voice problem, I could no longer practise as a non-specialist psychiatrist. To my delight, the niche role that was beginning to emerge fitted me much more perfectly than my traditional medical role ever had. Eventually, as I increased my hours and found ways to communicate despite my disability, I was given the opportunity to become a Senior Clinical Supervisor for the clinical and support staff at Buchanan Rehabilitation Centre.

Although I had to choose carefully what I said, as every word cost me significant effort, I enjoyed this role very much. It enabled me to contribute to the overall ethos and orientation of the newly-formed person-centred, recovery-focused unit. I was not doing any direct clinical work, but I was able to participate in the care of the staff and, through them, in the care and well-being of the people we were all there to serve. I loved getting to know the individual staff members I was supervising and appreciated the privilege of listening to them and learning from them. It was almost as if I was not in a 'role' at all but was simply being paid to be myself! What more could I ask?

Using the understanding that I had gleaned from my years of clinical work, research, training, and lived experience, I formulated a multimodal training course for all the staff at the hospital. I delivered the teaching in 12 weekly sessions. As the years went by, in groups of around eight per session, I taught the majority of the 60 staff the basic skill set. Everyone had the opportunity to practise the skills during the course as well as in their own lives. With technical assistance and helpful suggestions from others, I developed a series of dynamic PowerPoint slides, some of which were based on the original line drawings I had used in my research. This enabled us to develop a manual, with a copy for everyone. In this way, we created tools which were incredibly helpful to people in their work and in their lives. These were a compilation of everything I had learned. Staff were interacting with one another in the teaching sessions in a way that helped to create a trusting culture.

One of the slides was based on the spiral diagram that I had been developing since 1989 (see Figure 12.1 plus www.talkthatheals.org). An important contribution to my understanding of the recovery spiral had emerged from numerous telephone conversations with my best friend during that period in my life. We'd compare notes about the way life kept throwing up opportunities to have another go at things and to figure out how to re-cover old ground in new ways. She introduced me to the concept of 'victorious' cycles. The slide was cleverly animated to build up the picture of our life from birth to the current time and to show how we all re-cover the same old ground in our attempts to recover from the inevitable traumas and difficulties of life. It showed how vicious cycles can develop, and how each crisis can be viewed as an opportunity to create these victorious cycles by changing our thinking and choosing different actions. A spiritual, or meaning-making context, encompassed the spiral. In pairs, participants would place a picture of a physical bridge between them, and each person would consider their own re-covery journey. As they metaphorically built the Bridge of Trust, they told one another as much or as little of their own personal story as felt comfortable. They also practised actively listening to and validating one another.

Another essential tool and strategy I developed was the feelometer. In its original form, it was made from a substantial piece of strong cardboard covered in bright blue shiny paper with a smiley face at one end, a sad face at the other end and a neutral face in the middle. It had numbers from 0 (the worst you have ever felt) to 100 (the best you have ever felt) and a cursor that could be moved to identify how you feel at the moment. At the beginning of each group training session, I would pass the feelometer around the room to be used as a talking stick as we all continued to build the Bridge of Trust together.

'I'm feeling around 50 right now', I might say, 'because I didn't sleep all that well, and I'm a bit anxious about how we'll go today'. I would invite each person to identify *their* feelometer reading and say as much or as little about why they had chosen that percentage. We also used this ritual at the end of every session, writing names with before and after scores on the white board so that we could all see the changes that occurred. I always emphasised the importance of being honest, and we all agreed that there was no pressure and no judgment. Standing in a circle, we practised noticing and identifying one another's strengths (Rapp, 1998). We threw a soft teddy bear back and forth, picking out a person and naming things we appreciated about them:

'You are always on time.'
'You have a lovely smile.'

'Thanks for the cookies you baked.'
'You're willing to swap shifts at the drop of a hat.'

We practised identifying distressing thoughts and beliefs, and challenging them by asking whether this was true, or helpful, and what was the evidence? What might be a more helpful thing to tell ourselves? Together we learned to identify our thinking errors. My most common upsetting thought was: 'They'll think I'm stupid and they won't come next time'. Although it wasn't true, I guess this was a helpful thought to the extent that it made me more vigilant and careful to 'know my stuff', but as there was no evidence for it in the room, I found the list of thinking errors useful to name.

'Jumping to conclusions'; 'Fortune telling'; 'Catastrophising'. The more errors I could name, the better I would feel. This live demonstration of my own vulnerability gave others permission to be open too. Staff members found learning these skills particularly helpful in their personal lives. They often told me that they wanted more practice sessions.

The activity of 'being with' was taken up officially as a significant therapeutic intervention at Buchanan and could be recorded on the electronic data system for clinical notes. I developed an e-learning module to help staff understand more fully the way this could be put into practice. Special funding was made available for 'being with' activities. This meant support staff could now legitimately spend time as I had – maybe baking a cake with people, watching a movie or TV on the evening shift, or playing a game of cards. These activities were invaluable for building rapport and trust. It helped transform the hospital culture so that staff could feel that they did not always need to focus on 'observations', 'assessments', or 'problems', but also appreciate doing meaningful and fun activities together with the people they served. Undoubtedly many committed members of staff did such activities with people in their spare time. In the past custodial context, clinical and support staff were used to focusing on maintaining safety and being 'minders', often sitting in the staff room watching people through the window, or sitting with tick-charts 'monitoring' people. This was spirit breaking for everyone.

Each of the modalities included in the training could be recorded in the electronic notes in the same way as the 'being with' skills, to enable us to evaluate whether people who had received the training were using and recording the skills they had learned. This proved an effective way of creating feedback. It soon became apparent that staff who had done the training were applying their new skills in their clinical work as well as in their personal lives. There was a clear shift in values and attitudes, which was exciting to witness.

My feeling of joy increased. I was able to use my lived experience effectively, which gave me a different sort of authority. Sometimes I would joke that it was easier for me to sing than to talk, and if I was teaching a staff class, or speaking at a conference, I would briefly demonstrate a little operatic delivery of the point I was making. Fortunately, everyone was accepting and we all laughed together at my predicament. In retrospect, I wonder whether stopping the risperidone contributed to my regaining the capacity to feel joy.

Several years later (in 2005), a social-work student collected systematic feedback by interviewing all staff who had so far done the training. Staff described the training as helping them work more holistically and interact better with clients; to understand and be alongside them more. They described a change in their understanding of psychosis, an ability to identify vicious cycles and have more compassion. The training enabled them to communicate better in their personal relationships and manage their own stress as well as conflicts with their family members. They spoke of increased self-awareness and a sense of hope and meaning in their own lives. They said that with their colleagues, the shared model improved communication, supporting each other's work and validation of other clinicians. Separately surveying the clients revealed that they were appreciating staff 'being with' them and also helping them with self-reflection using the 'Map of Re-covery'.

Presenting these results over the following years at national and international conferences helped support an initiative that developed into recovery-oriented (and 're-covery') training for keyworkers and care coordinators in the community health centres around the greater Auckland region in New Zealand. Several hundred clinical staff received this training, which continued until the funding ceased in 2013. Pre- and post-evaluations continued to support the use of what eventually became known as the 'Re-covery Model', and the resources that we gradually developed and included for each clinician to take away.

Debbie and I went on to deliver similar training workshops for psychiatry registrars until my retirement in 2014. We invited the registrars to apply all these concepts to their own life journey. I also used the findings from the doctors-as-patients research that Josephine and I had been doing. I selected quotes from the study which the registrars read out in turn – a moving experience, putting themselves into the shoes of the participants, while opening doors for personal confidences to be shared safely in the group. The feedback we received was that they wholeheartedly appreciated and embraced our teaching. What always distressed us was that once they returned to their usual medical settings, they found it hard to put the recovery concepts and skills into practice because of the cultural pressures to conform.

Another pivotal moment in my own journey of recovery happened at the first southern hemisphere ISPS Symposium, held in Melbourne in 2003. Sitting next to Debbie, as psychologists John Read and Richard Bentall engaged in a debate with two psychiatrists about the impact of sexual abuse on the subsequent development of psychosis, I could not stop crying. I had made the connection between sexual abuse and my own experiences of psychosis, but to hear this link acknowledged in an academic setting was very powerful. These were tears of grief but also of relief and healing. On a subterranean level that

I had never reached before, I felt a deep sense of validation that somehow seemed to uplift and cleanse my soul. I held on to Debbie's hand, unable to speak. She seemed to understand.

That night, I had a dream. Buffy the dog had accidentally killed our Burmese cat, Yoko. Yoko, however, was not actually dead, although her body was in pieces (reminiscent of those jig-saw puzzle pieces that had repeatedly had meaning for me). Buffy was crying and saying 'I didn't mean to do it'. Was this some sort of premonition of what was to come? Much later, I painted a picture of this scene (see Figure 21.1).

As I was waking from this dream, I distinctly heard the words: *You are to be professor of psychiatry*.

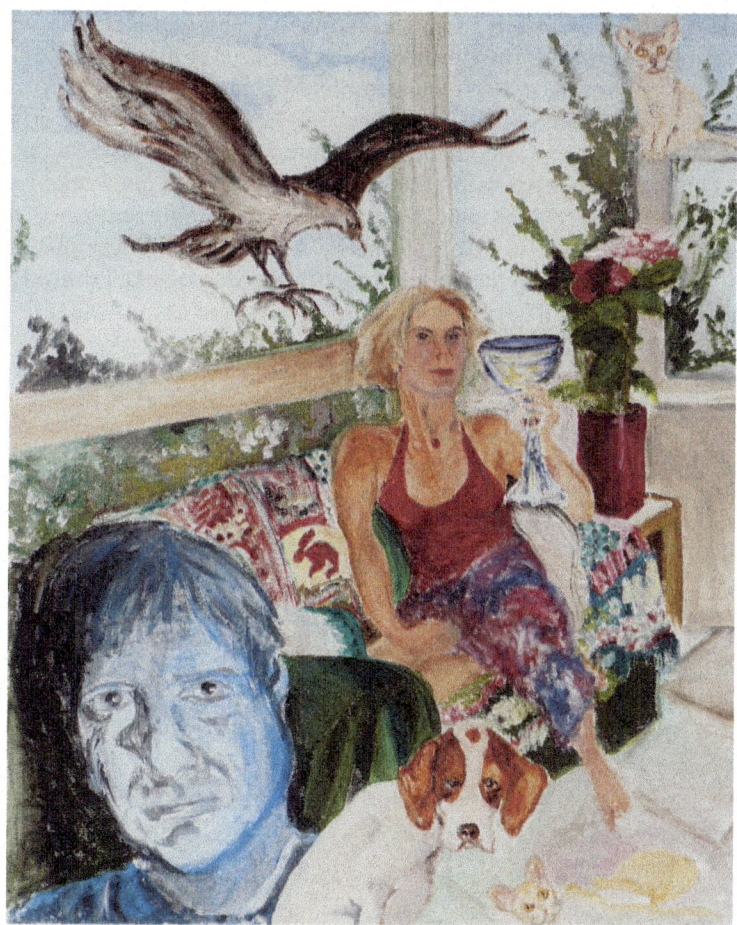

Figure 21.1 Painting of my dream.

This was so clear and stark that I said to Cam, 'I've just had the most extraordinary dream. It was like a voice telling me that I am to be professor of psychiatry'.

Cam didn't miss a beat. He immediately answered. 'Will I have to call you "Prof", or can I still call you Patte?'

It was such a lovely response! Usually he would react with concern to anything remotely outrageous that I might do or say. These humorous and accepting words were delightful to me. I'd never had an ambition to become a professor of psychiatry, but I wondered whether it might ever become a reality.

The rest of the conference was exciting and rewarding. At one point I found myself sitting next to Richard Bentall, cup of coffee in hand, telling him how his words had affected me, especially after what had happened to me in psychiatry. He told me he was glad to have met me and was very encouraging of my work. Once again, I felt included as part of the team of international contributors who were trying to make the world a safer place for people who experience psychosis. A group of us from New Zealand talked of forming a national branch of ISPS. This was to become an important peer group for me, as I became a committee member. Debra Lampshire later became our esteemed chairperson. Over subsequent years, I presented my work at annual *Making Sense of Psychosis* conferences in New Zealand, launched by our budding ISPS-NZ. As I went on to speak at ISPS conferences in England, Madrid, and Copenhagen, the people I met there became like family. But I'm running ahead of myself. There were more surprises to come.

22

DISRUPTION IN MEANING-MAKING
The Last Extreme State

In which Patte's seventh episode of psychosis overwhelms her family, and her recovery without 'antipsychotic' medication is received differently by different people.

It was spring 2003, some months after the Melbourne trip. My father-in-law was in the garden where I would usually find him on my return home from work. He was tending the new dahlias he had so patiently awaited as he did each year, the delicate orange and yellow shades of the new blooms gleaming in the late afternoon sun. These were an ancient species that had been transported from England by his forefathers, and he had faithfully dug up the tubers from his garden and replanted them when he moved to live with us ten years before.

We greeted one another and I went inside to make a cup of tea for us both, as I always did. Many conversations had been shared together over the years and we had enjoyed the closeness of our family bond. Sometimes we would pray together.

'Are you OK?' I asked, as he kicked his gumboots off at the door.

'No, actually', he said, wincing and holding his large life-worn hand loosely over his belly. I had noticed that he looked a little grey but now I could see clearly that he was in pain. He sat down, shaking his head.

'Sore tummy?' I asked. He nodded. Things moved quite fast from that moment. By late evening he had been admitted to hospital and a bowel obstruction was diagnosed. The next morning, he was recovering from emergency surgery. It was bowel cancer. Suddenly we were in the midst of a family crisis. I wanted to welcome him back to our home, which was, after all, his home too, and to support him if and when he could be discharged from the hospital. But I felt totally overwhelmed. I didn't realise how desperate I was feeling. I couldn't process it. For the first time in seven years I stopped sleeping and after a couple of nights I became very disturbed.

There is no way to get through this situation; whatever I choose feels unbearable. I must find a way out! I am crawling around the house

DOI: 10.4324/9781003153788-31

looking for some way to escape. Perhaps there is a hidden mouse hole that I can squeeze through. I am thinking of Truman in the movie 'The Truman Show'. I begin bowing to everyone and stepping backwards, reminiscent of when Truman finds the doorway out of the film set in which he has been trapped all his life. I am trying to find the handle of the door that will release me from this sad conundrum. I keep turning on my computer, expecting to see Richard Bentall. Surely, he will soon appear on the screen, ready to rescue me. (This was well before the days of Skype or FaceTime had even been invented. Much later I included a portrait of Richard in a painting depicting the images of the dream I had the day before meeting him at the Melbourne ISPS conference – see Fig. 21.1).

Cam wants me to go to hospital. I'll go because I know how hard it is for everyone right now. My best friend turns up, taking me aside to say it would be ridiculous for me to go to hospital. I slap her face, fearful that her words will destroy me and my family! She takes me out for a drive. All I can see are dead sheep standing in the fields at One Tree Hill Domain.

I realise that Cam must have been worried about me having another extreme state ever since I stopped the medication back in 2001. Why was his worst nightmare happening now? Now, when he was facing the possible death of his father. He needed me to support both him and his father, who I loved dearly. From his point of view, hospital was the best option. But my best friend knew so well how damaging hospital can be. She was aware of the risks, which were particularly acute for me, with my history of serious medication side effects. It was highly likely that in hospital, under the Mental Health Act, I would be given medication against my will. And yet I was willing to go to hospital if this was what my family needed. Sometimes, at its best, hospital can be a haven at such a time as this.

My friends and family came together to support us all. The crisis team arrived with home-visiting psychiatrists. I was committed under the Mental Health Act and, against all odds, they allowed me to stay at home with 24-hour nursing care. For some people, this committal process is a devastating, shaming experience, which makes recovery from extreme states even harder. For me, the experience was quite different. I have long thought of 'committal' as being the commitment of the mental health team to the person and their family. This is exactly how it felt, and I am grateful to everyone who was involved. My best friend contacted Debbie and they both spent the night alongside me. We spoke about it later as a 'pyjama party'. They helped me feel safe and accepted, sharing stories, and memories. We were able to laugh together.

Because of the serious side effects that I had repeatedly endured, a decision was made not to use 'antipsychotics'. I was prescribed only sedative pills, to help me sleep. What would have happened if I had been forced under the Act to go to hospital, and forced once again to take 'antipsychotic' medication? Thankfully I will never know.

That I was supported in this way was profoundly important in my recovery because it created a unique opportunity to find out whether this extreme state of psychosis would settle without 'antipsychotic' medication. To everyone's relief, not least my own, I slept well that night, and for the next few days I stayed on a small dose of anti-anxiety and sleeping medication. As always (at least as far as I saw it back then) I was back to my functioning self within a week. The Mental Health Act was allowed to lapse.

It was a remarkable revelation to me that I could indeed get through an extreme state such as this without recourse to 'antipsychotics'. To me it meant that, despite the fact that in these extreme states I had been 'as mad' as anyone I had ever 'treated' when I was in my psychiatrist role, I had probably never actually needed those toxic medications. All I seemed to need was something to help me sleep, and the support of my friends who were not fearful of my altered state but were prepared to 'be with' me. This discovery was to have a huge impact on my confidence in my ongoing capacity for mental health and my view of the future.

Following this episode, I was required by the Medical Council to see a psychiatrist, appointed by them, for an assessment of my fitness to practise. This was a voluntary undertaking on my part, but without it I would not have been awarded my practising certificate. Applying all my prior learning to my own situation, I developed a comprehensive recovery plan, which included an advance directive to make clear my preferences should another episode eventuate in the future. I was happy to put this in place to ensure safety in my professional role. It included a clear description of my early warning signs, such as an increase in feeling stressed and anxious, and not sleeping well for more than three days in a row. I detailed exactly what steps I would take should a similar pattern begin to emerge, such as who I would call, where I would go, and so on. Although at that time I did not fully understand the triggers, I knew my pattern of decompensation well enough to determine what was needed at the earliest warning signs. One action I took from that time was always to have some sedative medication in my bag that I could use if my anxiety levels became too extreme or if I didn't sleep. The pack of pills remains unopened 16 years later. It's about time I threw them away!

It is only now, looking back with the benefit of hindsight, I can see how this final extreme state arose. Despite our daily cups of tea, there had been an unresolved conflict between me and my dear father-in-law smouldering in the background over the months before he took ill. An extremely uncomfortable conversation had erupted while I was writing my paper on spirituality and psychosis. We had been talking about the concept of a 'spiritual emergency'. I was delighted to have the opportunity to explore and write about such a cutting-edge stimulating concept, as I saw it. I felt I was on the verge of a breakthrough which would help change the unremittingly pathologising paradigm usually applied to understanding psychosis. In my view, extreme states could be understood through the lens of a disruption in meaning-making, which could presage the emergence of a meaningful spiritual awakening. As I was explaining all this to my father-in-law, he had asked me a very provocative question.

'What if someone who has psychosis acts in dangerous ways that might harm a child? Shouldn't they then stay on medication?'

I was taken aback by his question. He had been aware that I was no longer taking medication because of my voice problem. As he told me more, I had found myself feeling increasingly upset. It transpired that for 17 years he'd held onto a 'memory' that he had never shared with me, from when my youngest son was five months old. He had witnessed my extreme state back then. I could hardly believe my ears as I heard him telling me that I had banged my baby's head on the wall.

He told me that I'd said, 'Mummy can bang your head if she wants to'.

At these surprising and bewildering words, shock, and horror had filled my senses. Spontaneously I cried out: 'That's not true!!'

I could not hold back my abhorrence at the thought of what he had just said. A sudden noise drew my attention to the back door. There, on the mat, a white dove lay dead. It was as if the pain we were both suffering had manifested itself in the form of this beautiful bird that often represents the Holy Spirit, lying lifeless before me. It felt like a spiritual emergency happening live.

I knew that my father-in-law must have been mistaken about what had happened. Neither did it fit with Cam's recollection nor that of the psychiatrist who had seen me during that time. What my father-in-law said made it sound, to my outraged and unbelieving ears, as if for all those years he had silently believed I had deliberately hurt my baby. In fact, quite the opposite was true. I had been hyper-vigilant, terrified that he might die because of my sense of being caught in the nuclear winter.

Recently I remembered that, prior to this final extreme-state episode, I had sought therapy in a bid to avoid these states happening again, now that I was no longer taking medication. During a therapy session, I brought up the subject of what my father-in-law had said to me. My new therapist encouraged me to imagine how I would like to respond to the upsetting words. In my fantasy interaction, I became so enraged with my father-in-law that I lost all control and ended up killing him. I didn't share the imagery with my therapist because I felt so horrified and shamed by it. In fact, in the session I dissociated and became withdrawn, quiet, and preoccupied. This meant I didn't receive the help from my therapist that might have assisted me in processing the unbearable emotions. I hadn't acknowledged them to myself, let alone to a therapist I barely knew.

Until writing this chapter, I could not understand why I was unable to resolve the situation with my father-in-law. Cam was caught in the middle.

We were in a kind of stand-off. I wanted him to convince his father that his memory was in error. We were never able to talk openly together about any of this. I'm wondering now whether the issue that had become so insurmountable in my mind was not the issue that really troubled Cam and his dad. Now I can see that Cam found himself in an impossible situation. He believed that I had an enduring mental illness, and that I needed medication to maintain my well-being. I wonder whether this was the issue that got in between us. It's only now that this realisation is falling into place. I feel so sad for the damage these unspoken concerns caused to my marriage and to my mental health.

Soon after the upsetting therapy session, I was faced with the possibility that my father-in-law's unexpected diagnosis of cancer either meant he might die, or that I might have to nurse him through his recovery. It felt unbearable to be in that situation and unbearable to be out of it. I could not find a way to accept him back into our home feeling so betrayed by my perception of his attitude to me, and I could not take a stand against him and refuse to take care of him in his hour of need. I needed a way out.

The intensity of those extreme emotions has echoes to this day, in the level of distress I experienced in response to Josephine's questions as we were writing this chapter. It's the closest we've come to abandoning the project of writing the book. I realise now that my father-in-law had no way of knowing the effect his question would have on me. I imagine that he was speaking on behalf of Cam, who no doubt had confided in him his ongoing concern about me remaining off medication. The paradox of what later unfolded strikes me as I write this. They wanted me to be on medication. Medication had caused me life-changing impairment. I had felt much better since stopping the medication. In a way, it was this unspoken conflict, caused by their *fear* about me not taking medication, that led to the final extreme state. The stigma of 'mental illness' being associated with dangerousness had found its way into my family and my home. It's as if I was no longer safe there. It is little wonder that I became psychotic. It makes sense that in my extreme state I was trying to find the exit from my life! I have come to believe that it is this type of emotional paradox that is the catalyst of my psychosis.

At the time that I was going through the extreme state back in 1987, when my youngest child was five months old, Jaakko Seikkula – a psychologist in Western Lapland – and his team were developing an approach called 'Open Dialogue' (Putman & Martindale, 2021). They would meet with the whole family at times of crisis, and skilfully give everyone a safe way to speak openly and be taken seriously. This resulted in less use of medication with great benefit to the person with psychosis, while also helping to heal rifts in the family. Josephine and I have often wondered how it would have been if my family had been able to access this approach back then. We could have talked about all the things that troubled each of us. Maybe I would not have endured further extreme-state episodes. Even in 2003, an open-dialogue approach might have enabled some very difficult and painful conversations to happen between me, Cam, and his father, which could have resolved years of hidden destructive tension. Open Dialogue was not available in New Zealand back then, nor is it still in 2021. In my view, as an effective evidence-based intervention, it should be used everywhere. It's about time.

Following my recovery, I felt strengthened by the knowledge of having come through this final extreme state without 'antipsychotics'. One day I asked Cam how he was feeling about what had happened during that last episode. It made me feel very sad to realise that, from his point of view, it had been an unmitigated 'nightmare'. He was working hard in all aspects of his life and just wanted life to feel 'normal', and to be able to enjoy our precious holiday times together. In retrospect, I can see how dreadfully unnerving and hopeless it must have felt for him. We had stability in our marriage for the six years that I was on risperidone. We had found peace together about the diagnosis of Bipolar Disorder. Now I was reviewing the whole thing once again. For Cam, the fact that I had not needed an 'antipsychotic' to get me through this acute situation did not help him to feel hopeful. He remained fearful that another episode could happen at any time. It was only years later that I found out that he held an unspoken fear that I might harm him in an altered state.

It was difficult for me to consider being on regular medication after so many toxic effects. I realise how fortunate I was to have been given the opportunity to learn to manage my life without it. I am aware that this is not an option for many people, for all sorts of different reasons. My voice was still as badly affected as ever, despite having stopped the risperidone, and indeed remained so for 12 more years. However, my life was feeling much better. My work was unfolding in a very satisfying way even with this disability and my perfect niche role was creating itself around me. It was as if, despite everything, God *was* going with me and giving me success, after all.

By the grace of God, my father-in-law survived the bowel cancer, and our relationship survived the vicissitudes of the next few months and years. He never returned to live with us but moved into a lovely supported home. Somehow, we remained loving friends until his death over ten years later. As he put it, he had been '93 times round the sun' by the time he left the planet. I like to tell people this when I am explaining the re-covery spiral! I visited him regularly and saw him the day before he died. His last words to me, accompanied by the most angelic smile, were: 'Here's beautiful Patte'.

That's grace!

23

LIGHTING A CANDLE FOR JUSTICE

In which Patte experiences a new sort of validation, and an ending.

In 2004, I was invited to run a workshop at the first Mental Health Spirituality and Wellbeing conference in Scotland. My best friend offered to accompany me. Presenting my ideas about spiritual emergency and my own lived experience of recovery felt exciting. After this, I was also scheduled to present a talk about my multimodal training course, at an ISPS conference in Manchester. I could hardly speak, but these opportunities were encouraging. Using a microphone and with silence in the room, I generally managed to be heard. Even the fact that my luggage did not arrive, and I had to wear borrowed clothes for my presentation in Dundee, did not deter me. It all went very well. It felt like I was on track.

And then another bomb dropped on top of me. The day after I had delivered my Dundee workshop, I received an email from Cam telling me that he had decided to leave me. He had already informed my mother of his decision, as he fully expected it might precipitate another episode of psychosis and he wanted her to be prepared. I was shattered. Except for the presence of my friend I would not have coped at all. She kept reminding me to 'look up', and to trust God. Her patient support, equanimity, and prayers in the face of my despair helped to get me through. We managed to travel to Manchester; I delivered my second presentation to the sound of appreciative applause; we visited my family and friends and received their commiseration and care, and we flew back to New Zealand.

Cam had moved out and was staying at a hotel. I sat in my rocking chair and sobbed my heart out, begging him to come home and 'try again'. Thankfully he agreed and we embraced as long-lost lovers might. Amazingly, we managed to find our way to a state of apparent tranquillity. Cam acknowledged that 'it was never a lack of love' that had torn him away, but just his fear about my instability and his concern that while I remained off medication I remained at risk, in his view. He confessed that he was fearful of what he perceived as my 'hostility' and worried that one day in an altered state I might harm him. At the time, I thought it was a ridiculous idea for him to have this fear of me. I now have much more compassion for his perspective, which mirrored his father's fears, carried silently over all those painful years, unbeknown to me. Since writing this book and facing the fact that I did indeed have unacknowledged murderous rage inside me, Cam's fears make even more sense.

A mutual friend recommended a book called *Fighting for Your Marriage* that she hoped might help us resolve our differences (Markman, Stanley, & Blumberg, 1996). We diligently worked on the exercises in the book, setting out for ourselves and one another our hopes, dreams, needs, and expectations for our marriage. My main issue was my felt need for Cam to 'recognise' me and validate me as someone who has strength and resilience and the capacity for wellness. I also wanted him to believe in me as someone who could make a contribution because of, rather than despite, my lived experience. People all over the world were starting to perceive me in this way but this was almost irrelevant in comparison. The only person I really wanted to 'see' me was Cam. All Cam wanted was peace and quiet, and to be able to enjoy his time off. We began to find ways of talking and listening to one another, and things seemed to be improving.

Eventually, we decided to look for a new home to mark the changes that we hoped were taking place. As we drove past our next-door neighbour's, he happened to be at his front door. We told him we were going to an auction. There and then, without any forewarning or foreknowledge, he said he would like to buy our house. Later that morning at the auction we bid for our new home. By the end of the day, we had bought a new house and sold our old one! It felt like flow. It seemed to me that we had turned a corner and that 'every day in every way, things were getting better and better'. We were working hard at repairing the damage that my extreme states had caused to the fabric of our marriage. I believed we were succeeding.

Our new home was delightful and our trips up to our holiday house in the Bay of Islands were becoming more romantic. We bought a flat for our two sons to live in; the older one was 22 by this time and the younger one was 18. Both were glad to 'leave home'. I began to trust that life was working out as I had always hoped, and I remembered my sentiments of almost 25 years previously when I first met Cam. *Could it be that all my dreams will be fulfilled with this young man?*

An odd little incident occurred one Saturday while we were sitting on the beach. Cam was stung by a wasp on his left ring finger. His finger began to swell; his wedding ring was restricting the circulation. We drove urgently to the local hospital. As a casualty doctor, Cam had been required to use wire cutters to remove rings in similar circumstances. He ended up having to cut his own wedding ring off his finger while I sat in the car waiting for him, wondering what was taking so long.

Around this time, a couple of friends encouraged me to speak to a confidential forum that the New Zealand government had set up for people who had concerns regarding mental health services before 1990. This was in recognition of the fact that prior to 1990 there had been no complaints process. I wondered whether it might be an opportunity to tell my story to the judge. At last it might be possible to shed some light on what had happened back in 1989, when I was thrown out of the psychiatry training scheme.

Cam did not want to accompany me so I went alone. It was a Friday, 4 November 2005. Sitting in front of the committee, my heart pumping, I found words to describe what had occurred. The judge took my copies of the 'evidence', including the letter from the professor who had chaired the training committee and those written spontaneously in my defence by my supervisors, contesting his words. When I had finished speaking, Judge Anand Satyanand (who later became the Governor General of New Zealand) said: 'I'm lighting a candle for you to get justice'.

He gave me the name of an employment lawyer who he advised me to consult, and a tape recording of the session. I went home feeling a sense of relief and joy. Hugging Cam, I asked him to listen to the tape recording with me. His tone was serious and sad when he responded that he might listen to it on his own some time but did not want me to be there. I was dumbstruck. All I really wanted was for Cam to be able to join with me in seeing what had happened from my point of view, but it seemed impossible for him.

In trepidation, the next morning I said to Cam that if he still wanted to leave me, now was the time to go. By the Sunday he had left. Three weeks later he was dating the woman from his work with whom he had always had a bond. She had separated from her husband a year earlier. By then, they had worked together for 20 years.

24

WAYS OF MAKING SENSE

In which Patte experiences a series of meaningful co-incidental events, rekindling her sense of pathway and purpose in life.

My worst nightmare was being manifest. But somehow, on some level, I accepted it. I believed Cam when he told me that his new romantic liaison was not the underlying reason for him leaving, but I also knew she had always been there in the background the whole time he had been working in his General Practice. I thought back to the repeated anxious 'voice' I had heard over the previous years which had said that Cam would have an affair.

It was now a reality. Miraculously, I felt protected from the full blast of the devastation of it all. Maybe not so strangely, I found myself feeling less lonely in solitude than I had when alongside my beloved husband who acknowledged that he could not understand me or believe in me. Even though I had ample cause to feel enraged, the hostility ebbed away, leaving me with an uncanny peace. One morning soon after, lying in bed alone, I 'heard' the words: *Know that you are very loved.*

This was not an audible voice in my ears but a still small voice in my heart. I felt held by an invisible love that pervaded and surrounded me, despite my circumstances. The next day the words, *Know that you are forgiven,* impressed themselves on my inner being, reassuring me that I was forgiven for everything that had happened. Forgiven for the effects that the extreme states had on my life, on my marriage, and on the lives of my loved ones. Forgiven for the effects that taking the medication had on my brain and my voice. And I knew I needed to forgive Cam. He was walking away from 25 years of our investment in one another and our marriage. He was walking away from everything we had built together, and the hope of a bright and loving future as we grew old together. And now I was alone in our beautiful big house with our two beautiful big dogs that we had chosen together, and that had helped to bond us in so many ways. The reality of it all was unbearably painful to contemplate. It was a situation that I would never have chosen for myself. I wrote in my prayer diary:

DOI: 10.4324/9781003153788-33

Lord, I can't take any more pain. I need to know your loving arms are around me, whatever happens next.

Later that day, putting on my trainers and accompanied by my two aristocratic dogs, I trudged around the park thinking of all the future situations that were likely to unfold now that Cam and I were apart. Sadness and anger filled my broken heart. Almost at the end of my walk, I noticed an auburn-haired young man coming towards me. I recognised him as Mark, the son of some friends from church. He had a black dog with him. Suddenly my two dogs lunged forwards. I was holding onto their leads tightly in my left hand, so I was automatically pulled to the ground by their unexpected movement. Crack! I felt a searing pain in my hand. On my knees, clutching my injured hand to my chest, the floodgates broke open and uncontrollable sobs wracked my body. Within seconds, warm comforting arms enfolded me.

'Thank you, Mark', I mumbled, so grateful for human contact from this young friend at such a time of grief and pain. My prayer of a few hours previously flashed into my mind, and I was thanking God too, profoundly consoled by the sense of an answer. It was as if God's divine loving arms were holding me in a heavenly embrace.

'That's OK', said an unfamiliar voice, 'but my name is James'.

I looked up through my tears into the handsome, youthful face of a total stranger who was clasping me tightly and looking at me with concern in his kind eyes. We untangled ourselves and I laughed, explaining my mistake, and thanking him again. I reassured him that I would be OK. He reluctantly let go of me, gathered up the escaped dogs, and we went our separate ways.

In our working on this chapter, Josephine expressed the worry that people might think that I believed God listened to my prayer and brought this man to hold me. As I took on board her concerns, I realised that it would never have occurred to me that people would think like that. I do not have a literal way of seeing God as a kind of Santa Claus in the sky who sends 'answers to prayers' in that way. For me, this sequence remains a much more mysterious lived experience and I am comfortable with not knowing how these synchronous events come about. I just accept that experiences like this are *real* in terms of how they *feel* for me when they happen, and I am grateful for them.

But Josephine's comments prompt me to describe more of what happened when I felt the young man's arms around me. It was a literal 'holding', but it felt way beyond the physical holding. There was something powerful about it that linked with the words that I had written in my prayer journal that morning, explicitly stating that I needed to know 'your loving arms are around me'. It was even more meaningful because it was a stranger's arms around me, not the arms of my young friend. This was so unusual in my experience – to have a total stranger, a man around 30 years my junior, embracing me with kindness and comfort, which is what I so needed at that moment. There was meaning for me beyond the details of the incident; a sense of 'I am held', that 'all will be well'.

Unlike my mother as a nine-year-old saying, 'If there *is* a God, "he" doesn't care about me' – in my case this was a lived experience that indicated that if there is a God, 'he' *does* care about me. It's a total mystery as to how these things happen. What matters is the meaning I experience in the moment. If anything, this specific experience brings to mind Yeshua, the young Jewish man who, 2,000 years ago, became known amongst his followers for the power of his loving presence, which went way beyond their everyday expectations.

To continue with the story, sure enough, I had broken a bone in my left hand; the metatarsal of my ring finger had snapped in two! So just as Cam had needed to remove his wedding ring from his finger six months previously, I now was forced to remove my wedding ring from mine.

Despite the initial relief I had fleetingly felt that our conflicted marriage appeared to be over, within days of this accident I thought I heard the still small voice telling me: *As your hand heals, so shall your marriage be healed.* And then, *After the adultery Cam will return and you will accept him back.*

Subsequently, I had the expectation that Cam would be back within six weeks as my hand healed. Oddly I did not miss him. I certainly did not relish the idea of accepting him back after the affair. Even so, I passionately wanted to believe that our marriage would be saved. Then, a series of events left me believing that I was meant to wait for Cam to return. I happened to meet a relative of his at the wedding of a friend. She told me that she was praying that Cam's new romantic relationship would 'turn to gravel in his mouth'. I was surprised to hear these sentiments, as the idea of praying something like that seemed a bit 'unchristian' to me. I had no idea it was a scripture.

The next day, my best friend told me she had just been reading Proverbs 20:17. It said that 'stolen bread tastes sweet but soon turns to gravel in the mouth'. Another coincidence! Now I could understand what Cam's relative was saying. Cam's romantic affair was 'stolen bread'. It was like a reassurance. If the whole affair turned to gravel in his mouth, it would be a lot easier to accept him back. I would have been so jealous and hurt at the idea that he loved that woman more than he loved me.

I wanted my marriage to last forever. I hoped that, together, our love would grow and reap the benefit of our years of hard work. The idea of the affair turning to gravel in his mouth kept me hoping that Cam and I would get back together. On one occasion he asked if he could talk with me, but I did not feel ready to hear what he had to say. I knew that the relationship had not yet turned to gravel in his mouth. And six weeks passed, but he did not return. It felt so meaningful to me that my best friend had been reading the same phrase as Cam's relative had prayed. It kept me going. I was prepared to wait as long as it took.

Several weeks later, another memorable sequence of coincidences had an even more powerful impact on my sense of well-being. It was time to take the big next step of setting up my own separate bank account, a symbol of my unwanted singledom. Having a coffee with a friend just prior to going to the bank, I was distraught. Tears of intense sadness and regret filled my eyes. Despite my hopes, this seemed so final.

As it happened, my friend and I had recently both read Eckhart Tolle's book, *A New Earth* (Tolle, 2005). It told a story about a king who had every worldly possession and yet was repeatedly experiencing terrible sadness. He called all the wise men from his kingdom together to ask their advice to help him get through his unbearable distress. If they could help him, he would give them half his kingdom. One old sage brought the king a gold ring which he should never remove from his finger. Whenever the king experienced intense sadness, he was to read the words inscribed around its circumference: *This too will pass*. It was the first time I had ever heard that phrase.

Seeing my pain, my friend took my hand. 'Remember the book', she said. 'This, too, will pass'.

As we left the café on our way to the bank, we bumped into another friend of mine, Jeffrey Masson. I hadn't seen him for several months and he did not know about Cam's departure. He asked how I was, and I briefly caught him up with my unhappy situation.

Jeffrey then said: 'Well, you know, my father had a ring, and on that ring were written the words, 'This too will pass'. It's a very useful phrase to remember when things feel really bleak'.

The juxtaposition of these two identical reminders coming to me from independent sources had a profound effect. It was as if the meaning of the words was galvanised in my soul. I felt as if I had almost physically been given a protective shield; a comforting shawl of words to wrap around me in my times of grief and pain. Over the years since then, this simple phrase has frequently protected me from despair at times of suffering.

That it was Jeffrey who was part of this synchronicity is so multi-layered for me. He had written the highly publicised and controversial book, *The Assault on Truth: Freud's Suppression of the Seduction Theory* (Masson, 2003). His argument was that Freud had initially believed that the 'conversion' symptoms suffered by his patients were caused by sexual abuse in early childhood, but he was reluctant to face the reality of such a shocking finding. Fearful of public reaction, as well as rejection from the medical establishment, Freud instead attributed his patients' descriptions of their experiences to 'fantasy'. In 2005, I was only just beginning to understand the role that my own childhood experiences had played in my extreme states, in what had happened to me in my psychiatry training, and in the eventual breakdown of my marriage. It is poignant to reflect now on my mother's dismissal of my 11-year-old attempts to tell her about my experiences in the light of the influence that Freud's theories had on her generation. Now we all know so much more about the deleterious effects of childhood sexual abuse than anyone did back then. As I think back, with 2020 hindsight, I wonder too about the dream-like significance of the gold rings in this series of synchronicities. First, the loss of Cam's wedding ring, then of mine, and finally, the references to the inscribed ring with the wise reminder that 'this too will pass'.

How I make sense of what happens in my life is pivotal to my sense of well-being. I still find an open-hearted fascination for the mystery of the experience of meaning in the unfolding of events. Sometimes the hope inspired by these juxtapositions is what makes life feel most worth living.

Cam eventually let me know in an email that he would never want to return to the marriage. At that time, I refused to believe him. And yet in retrospect, I can see that he meant it. Now 15 years have gone by and he is content with his life, albeit with its ups and downs. Our sons quickly accepted the fact that we were a divided family. They told me that they believed I was better off for it, and therefore they were too. It turns out that they were right. They maintain a close connection with their father, and Cam and I want only the best for one another. I no longer have any desire for his relationship with the woman who replaced me to turn to gravel in his mouth. I am glad he has her in his life.

Another question I ask myself now is what would have happened if I had remained on the risperidone, or some other dopamine-blocking 'antipsychotic' medication that might have prevented me from perceiving that heightened sense of meaning-making that got me through all this? I guess it's possible that the marriage would have survived, and I would have lived a toned-down existence where the colours were never as bright as before. Would that have been better than what actually happened? I doubt it. And how would I have coped in the years following the break-up if I had known that Cam would never return? I can only be thankful for the severe mercy of having believed that the marriage would be restored.

25

THE RE-COVERY MODEL

In which Patte receives validation in international contexts and locally, using her lived experience, learning and ideas collaboratively with others, finding hope and new possibilities. Hope can be found in the lived experience of psychosis.

After the confidential forum, before I broke my hand, I met with the lawyer recommended to me by the judge. Thinking that going to court might be the right way forward, I told her what had happened. The lawyer – a feisty woman several years younger than me – listened to my story with interest and concern. A full-on court case might unleash another wave of stigma and discrimination, she warned me. Her suggestion was to get a report from my psychiatrist and seek some sort of restorative justice. As I heard her reflect on my situation, I realised that I wanted and needed to get my power back. I could understand her perspective but I wanted to be more proactive on my own behalf, rather than simply relying once again on the so-called experts to give their assessment of my mental health.

I had recently received a newsletter from the District Health Board with a link to an article describing the impact and value of my work. My ideas and theoretical frameworks were out in the world. The people who had tried to disqualify me needed to see this. They couldn't deny that the reasons they used, when they did not reappoint me all those years before, were clearly spurious; indeed, they were wrong. If I were to get my psychiatrist to write a report, I wanted to be part of the team. I decided to ask a number of my senior colleagues, including my psychiatrist and the Medical Council psychiatrist, to line up alongside me to present my case to the old guard. I didn't want retribution; I just wanted everyone to be on the same page about what had happened. I wanted to arrange a meeting with the original training committee members so I could demonstrate that my ideas and theoretical frameworks were being embraced locally and globally. I wanted them to see, too, that I was thriving in terms of my mental health, despite the impact of their harmful

DOI: 10.4324/9781003153788-34

decision 16 years previously. Then they would see they had made a huge mistake. I wanted an apology.

Fired up with enthusiasm, I sent off an email detailing my request. It makes me smile as I write this, to think of what might have happened if we had taken my plan forward. The image from my extreme state in 1989, of me flying the plane with the whole of the psychiatric fraternity on board, comes to mind. I once told a therapist about this vision. She asked me how I had managed to get everyone onto the plane. After thinking about it for a few seconds, I said, 'I must have forced them'. My therapist had pointed out that, 'God does not use force'. This had given me pause for thought. I didn't want to force people to see things my way. It probably would have been a fiasco. Fortunately, because I sent the email just before Christmas, it gave me time to review my situation. By the New Year, I realised that I didn't want to take this avenue after all, especially because by then my marriage was in deep trouble, and I needed all my energy to focus on my own well-being.

Eventually, however, in recognition of what I had requested, the Medical Council psychiatrist sent me a draft report that he was preparing for the Medical Council. He encouraged me to make corrections to it if need be. In the report, he wrote about my recovery journey and acknowledged my wellness. He stated that my diagnosis had been Brief Psychotic Episodes, not Bipolar Disorder, and there was no further requirement for me to report to the medical council or to see a psychiatrist. He also spelled out the contribution I was making to recovery training – nationally and internationally. I was very grateful to him. It gave me the confidence to proceed.

Over the following years, several senior colleagues urged me to complete my registration to become a fully qualified psychiatrist, but by this time I had well and truly decided that I did not want to do this.

Writing that email to my senior colleagues helped me formulate my forward plan. This became the jumping-off point for the next initiative in telling my story in a new way. In the global recovery movement, people such as Laurie Curtis often said that 'recovery is not a model, it's an experience'. I wanted to make it clear that the 'Re-covery Model' provided a framework for clinicians to put the recovery approach and principles into practice. And what better way to show this than by using the authority and credibility of my own lived experience!

In 2006, a presentation I submitted for the ISPS congress in Madrid was chosen as one of a series of special lectures to celebrate their 50th anniversary. For my work to be acknowledged in this way felt exciting. This was the first time I used the 'Re-covery Model' to tell my story publicly. Sitting on the stage with a colleague interviewing me, I began by answering questions about the extreme state that happened in 2003. Then we worked back from my early life, painting a verbal and pictorial description of events. My colleague was demonstrating my model, and I was talking about my life as she showed how to put the model into practice.

I explained how the patterns and triggers developed, and how I had become aware that in fact I did not have a chronic, relapsing psychotic illness, or mood disorder, but rather the ongoing effects of repeated traumatic experiences. I acknowledged that there had been a lot of grief and anger to deal with, and I had to learn to tolerate the intensity of my own distress, which was probably the hardest thing. At the end of the talk, we came back to the beginning and I talked about how I got through the final episode without medication; such a triumph for my recovery!

The lecture was a great success. Ann-Louise Silver came up to thank me afterwards. She was one of the pioneering therapists in the Chestnut Lodge research, which had been mistakenly reported to indicate that psychotherapy was not helpful for people with diagnoses of schizophrenia (McGlashan, 1984). Ann-Louise knew from her own experience how valuable their approach had been. She told me that it was especially poignant for her to hear me speak, with my hardly audible voice, as it so emphasised the importance of the work we were all doing to develop the use of psychological support rather than the use of medication. I was moved. Yet again, I felt as if I was being accepted into the fold amongst therapists and clinicians who had spent their lives trying to improve the care offered to those who, like me and the people I serve, had endured psychotic states.

Later in the morning, I attended another special lecture by Malcolm Stewart, a psychologist who also came from Auckland but who I did not know at that time. As I listened to Malcolm's lecture, which was about why it is useful to have a *shared model* in psychiatry, I resonated strongly with the rationale that he was putting forward. He was describing his own stress/vulnerability/strengths model in this context. At the end of his talk, he mentioned me.

'I've just heard Patte Randal's special lecture and actually her "Re-covery Model" is even more integrative than mine'.

After the lecture, I thanked him for his surprising acknowledgement. I asked whether he would be interested in writing a paper with me, putting forward his rationale for the importance of having a shared model, along with the 'Re-covery Model', as a model that met all the advantages he had described. Malcolm immediately agreed. It took several years but by 2009 we had published a paper in the newly established ISPS journal, *Psychosis* (Randal et al., 2009). It felt like an achievement to have more of my ideas and theoretical models published.

Prior to 2001, before my brain was damaged by the risperidone, I would always read out my presentations at conferences. However, my voice impairment made reading aloud almost impossible. As I continued to teach my multimodal training course in various university settings, my best friend, herself a doctor, helped me present my story using the 'Re-covery Model'. She had contributed the concept of 'victorious cycles', so it seemed fitting for us to be presenting together in what became such a victorious cycle for me.

179

Speaking spontaneously was slightly easier than reading aloud. In the end, I no longer needed notes. I did not believe I'd ever be able to return to a clinical role, but I continued to supervise and teach staff. However, with practice, I was gradually gaining confidence in using my limited voice.

Although I was regularly speaking about my lived experience at conferences, I had never shared my personal story face to face with the people I served. Using everything I had learned from Debra Lampshire, I now had the opportunity to make all that I was teaching to the staff at Buchanan Rehabilitation Centre accessible to the residents, and to go even further. I explained that my strange-sounding voice was a side effect of medication. I let everyone know that I had experienced psychosis and recovery myself. This was revolutionary for me, but it was a natural evolution. I had eventually found a way to be able to contribute to my clinical work from my experiences of extreme states. Here was a perfect context for me to begin to disclose limited aspects of my own lived experience, for the first time, to the people I served. I began to run what I called 'Beliefs Groups', which were based on Debra's groups, but integrated the use of the 'Re-covery Model'.

Both staff and residents were invited to join the new style groups, including psychiatry registrars and other psychiatrists. These were much appreciated, with consistent positive feedback from everyone. I used examples of how my own psychotic thinking had come about. I would describe in detail, using the five-part model, the sequence that led to my belief that I was in the nuclear winter. This was an application of 'therapeutic use of self' but was also taking an educational recovery-focused approach. It was in one of these sessions that the young man pointed out to me that what had happened to me must have been worse than a nuclear winter. He taught me something invaluable. The lovely thing about these groups was the reciprocity. As we built the Bridge of Trust, we would all contribute our lived experience so that we could learn from one another.

I used my PowerPoint presentation, made into booklets that everyone could keep, which demonstrated the 'Re-covery Model' and all the skills we were learning, including a list of thinking errors. It is important not to directly challenge so-called psychotic delusional beliefs, or indeed any strongly held beliefs, because this tends to entrench them even further.

What I was teaching people to do in these groups was to get to a place of trust where we would disrupt our own beliefs and figure out our own thinking errors. I would always share my own distressing beliefs, as I had in the staff training groups. For example, I might write something on the whiteboard that was bothering me such as:

I always have to get things right, otherwise no one will respect me.

The more thinking errors I could notice in this sentence, the better I would feel, and my feelometer score would go up. So, in a way, the more I could identify what I got *wrong*, the better the outcome for me! This self-disclosure made us all laugh. It also made it safe for others to follow suit. In our groups, we only looked at the errors in thoughts which made us feel worse. We didn't address thoughts that made us feel better, however 'delusional' those sorts of thoughts may have been. There was nothing confronting, insulting, or critical in these sessions. Everyone was mutually respectful, supportive, and validating.

As a teacher, by using the 'Re-covery Model' to disrupt my own vicious cycle patterns, I was showing everyone how to disrupt theirs; I was leading the way through the process, towards victorious cycles. Eventually, the young people who attended these sessions decided to call them 'Understanding Ourselves Groups', because it was clear to them that the outcome was an increase in personal understanding. I loved this role as educator and tutor.

I became increasingly confident being back in my clinical role again, even with my voice disability. Eventually, I once again took on a role as a non-specialist psychiatrist, even prescribing medication when necessary. Using the 'Re-covery Model' to work collaboratively with individuals, I helped them understand the impact of what had happened to them, culminating in their hospital admissions and the subsequent need to be at the rehabilitation centre. I was always surprised when people elected to stay on 'antipsychotics', even when I offered them the opportunity to safely decrease the doses. It was a reminder to me that I needed to be guided by each person as they figured out what works for them.

These were exciting times for me, sharing knowledge and challenges in a collaborative educational way. I wanted to take this educational stance further. By 2007, recovery colleges were emerging in England. These are educational facilities, set up initially by clinicians with lived experience of recovery sharing the knowledge and skills acquired. Now, in the UK and Europe, dozens of these colleges are offering hundreds of mental health, well-being, and recovery courses co-designed and co-delivered by peers together with clinicians. These courses and workshops include: how to deal with difficult emotions, mindfulness skills, goal-setting, interview skills, healthy living, and listening and communication skills. They have been taken up by thousands of people, including peers, family members, clinical staff, and the wider community, with significant benefit (Crowther et al., 2019; Toney et al., 2018). Back in those early days, I floated the idea of Buchanan Centre becoming New Zealand's first Recovery College. This never became a reality but I was encouraged one day when I was walking to the local shops to get my lunch. I passed a young woman with her friend. She greeted me with a big smile.

'There's my teacher!' she said to her friend.

I suddenly recognised her as a participant of the 'Understanding Ourselves' group from several years before. At the time she had been struggling with severe life issues and extreme states. I asked what she was doing now.

'I'm studying journalism', she told me proudly.

We parted with a warm sense of achievement – her, for obvious reasons; and me, because I realised that in her experience, my vision of creating a Recovery College had almost been a reality. I think even now, my ideal would be to co-create training opportunities, offering a hybrid of life and well-being skills and educational support which becomes self-perpetuating. But more of this is given in Chapter 26.

Around that time, Debbie returned from a conference in England where she had acquired a set of prompt cards to identify 'early warning signs' presented by psychologist Jo Smith. These depicted changes in thoughts, feelings, and actions. I modified this set to include a set of 'body sensations' cards, and then arranged the cards by colour-coding to fit into the five-part model. The cards demonstrated how everything interacts with everything else, often in a vicious cycle. As we began to use them in routine clinical practice, a clever, articulate young man called Joel made a comment.

'We need more cards. We need cards to help us name all the things we can't yet understand about our patterns'.

This observation precipitated a new era at the rehabilitation centre. We asked a group of young people who had been attending our groups to join us in a working party to co-create the requested prompt cards. We brainstormed all the aspects of the 'Re-covery' journey we needed to know about in order to create victorious cycles, rather than being continually stuck in vicious cycles. We were actively and mindfully examining our thinking, our feelings, our body sensations, and our actions in all phases of what we'd each been through. It was wonderful to be with one another in such a collaborative, creative way. After many focused weeks, we ended up with the following six priceless sets of cards (including some additional ideas gleaned from already existing tools such as one identifying medication side effects (Day et al., 1995), but modified to fit the colour-coded approach):

When I'm at my best
Ways of getting support and things that help when I'm not so good
What are my triggers and what makes me vulnerable?
What are my early warning signs?
What side effects of medication do I experience?
What are my risk behaviours and thoughts?

Soon we began to use the cards to help collaboratively identify patterns that could populate the recovery plans that were required to be formulated as part of best practice. These plans included a page for each card set. Instead of prompt cards for the positive effects of medication, we included a page to facilitate a brainstorm with each person about the ways in which medication was helpful in creating a victorious cycle, in terms of changes in body sensations, feelings, thoughts, and actions for each individual. I was always impressed by how clear people were about these things. Over the ensuing several years, I personally worked individually with over 50 young people (aged between 17 and 50) to collaboratively develop their 'Re-covery' plans. Everyone was then able to take their own 'plan' with them on discharge. Often these plans would be used to help the person advocate for themselves in terms of getting optimal use of medication, if it was needed, or support with reducing it, or ensuring that they had access to those facilities and resources that helped them maintain a victorious cycle.

This was extremely rewarding work. It would sometimes take three months of weekly sessions to complete this collaborative effort. On many occasions, people subsequently went through more 'rounds' of their 're-covery' patterns, manifesting further episodes of psychosis. Initially I felt I'd failed when this happened, but we soon discovered that reflection on this next episode enabled them to become more aware of their patterns. It's as if they needed another round to consolidate their learning. In retrospect, I can see that it had been the same for me. Many of the young people left the rehabilitation centre well equipped with that knowledge. Each crisis was viewed and experienced by the person and the staff as another learning opportunity to help create future victorious cycles; a paradigm shift in thinking about extreme states.

With the tools I had developed, I was routinely able to complete this brief focused intervention in around 12-hour-long sessions. This was in contrast to the 200 hours over two years that I had devoted to supporting the participants in my research study. Most of the people I was working with currently had also attended at least one eight-week course of 'Understanding Ourselves' groups. Time was spent more efficiently and effectively than in my early research days.

These things became part of what the service offered. Several young people had come to the centre with diagnoses of so-called schizophrenia, apparently enduring 'symptoms' and 'hopeless' prognoses. When the time came for them to leave Buchanan Rehabilitation Centre, they were pursuing their hopes and dreams, venturing into the peer workforce, attending university, or entering careers. On more than one occasion, a young person presented their own recovery story alongside me or another clinician, at a grand round or ISPS conference, using the 'Re-covery Model' as a framework for making sense of their journey. This was not an early intervention (Yung et al., 1998). This was a late intervention, and it was working. Together we were finding hope in the lived experience of psychosis.

My ideas and theoretical frameworks were being validated in so many ways – at international conferences; the publication of my model; and hundreds of people being trained in my method via the key-worker, care-coordinator and registrar trainings, and in other settings. I was invited to teach a number of university courses. The 'Re-covery Model' now has a life of its own and is being taught without me.

In 2011, *Experiencing Psychosis: Personal and Professional Perspectives* – a book that I had been invited to coedit and co-author along with Jim Geekie, Debra Lampshire, and John Read – was published in the ISPS series (Geekie,

Randal, Lampshire, & Read, 2011). The theme was how we go about the business of understanding and relating to the subjective experience of psychosis. Chapters written by ten contributors with experience of different aspects of these states – such as hearing voices, existential loss of self, negative symptoms, or delusional beliefs – were paired together with chapters written by contributors who had done research into those same aspects of lived experiences. A paradigm shift in meaning-making was happening. We had a book launch at the Women's Bookshop in Ponsonby. The room was full. Standing around looking gorgeous in our glad rags, we toasted one another with glasses of bubbly. When Jim Wright, my old friend and mentor, my one-time nemesis, came to join the celebration and brought his lovely daughter – who is also a psychiatrist – along with him, I felt we had come full circle. It was the icing on the cake for me.

26

LIVING THE EXPERIENCE OF NOW
My Life Beyond Psychiatry

In which Patte tentatively ventures to hope that the fulfilment of dreams of a lifetime are becoming a reality.

As with everyone's life, mine is full of the minutiae that make up the day. I sit here in my home in Raglan, New Zealand, where I moved two years ago. After I purchased this house, I discovered that this glorious sea-side Shangri-La was designated New Zealand's most beautiful small town that year. From the moment I moved in, I've felt at home. Like most of the world, I am enduring the aftermath of the Covid-19 crisis. So far, it has been a mixed experience, initially providing focused writing time under lockdown, here in my own personal slice of Heaven. Latterly, I have noticed times of loneliness and isolation, feeling far from family and friends in England and America. I have become extremely thankful for Skype and Zoom, and I am sure I'm not alone in that. For now, the internet is our much-appreciated gift for keeping us all connected at this unprecedented time, with the problems of climate change thrown in. The vision that I saw back in 1988 comes to mind.

It is a scene from the future. Devastation. Old and new cars litter the roadside, unable to be used. No air travel is possible. There is danger, a sense of emergency and catastrophe. My oldest son is a man, living overseas and I 'know' I will never see him face to face again except via some form of electronic communication on a screen. He and my brothers are creating a computer programme to save the world.

I'm not sure about the computer programme to save the world, but who knows!?

My desk overlooks the estuary and jagged Mount Karioi, a 2.4-million-year-old volcano. Sitting here at my computer, I can see the teal blue of the sky reflected in the sea as the tide creeps in. There are bright weeping willows swaying in the breeze, and the resonant tones of a tui accompany me, while a

DOI: 10.4324/9781003153788-35

sacred kingfisher flashes gold and turquoise as he dives from the manuka tree. Gazing at the dark outline of the mountain, I'm reminded of these words:

> I lift up my eyes to the hills. From whence does my help come? My help comes from the Lord, who made Heaven and Earth.

I find myself asking for help as various challenges arise day by day. Thankfully, somehow, the help I need makes itself available one way or another. I continue to be grateful for the provision I receive.

I'm 69 years old and retired from clinical work, although still pursuing my passion, integrating all I have learned into 'The Gift Box', a practical resource for supporting mental health and well-being (see Chapter 30). My life remains full of delightful people of all ages whose company I treasure. I do not miss my 'work'. For the final 14 years of my employment, I was always aware of the privilege of being paid to be myself. I suppose, in some ways, I'm still being paid to be myself. I receive superannuation and because of my good fortune I have no need to work for more income. A simple life is all I want – walking with my little 14-year-old dog, Oscar; writing; playing my ukulele and singing with the band of friends who call ourselves 'The Jammies'; dancing or Zumba in the town hall for exercise; meeting friends for coffee or the occasional lunch in the café that overlooks the glorious sea view downtown. My house was built on poles in the late 70s and has a self-contained flat below. It's a classic Kiwi bach, and my sons love coming to stay, along with their partners. My friends do too!

In the past 18 years since 2003, I have managed to maintain ongoing victorious cycles in my life journey without further episodes of psychosis. I have remained off all medication. I no longer see myself as having had Bipolar Disorder. My view is that I endured many extreme states at times when life became too painful and didn't make sense. My meaning-making system went into overdrive, tipping up the jigsaw puzzle for me to see the dream-like pieces scattered around. Now it is possible to put them together and make sense of what happened so much more coherently. Everything has fallen into place. It's interesting, reflecting on all this with the benefit of hindsight. Even when we are on the right path, we don't necessarily know it. It's just a matter of plodding on. Maybe that is what people mean by the dark night of the soul. And sometimes there is an intense sense of purpose. For me, each of these extremes was, in a sense, a 'spiritual emergency' through which I gradually discovered a solid, reliable loving foundation. A feeling of purpose and meaning enriches my life, underpinned by having made sense of what I have been through and suffered.

There are times when I feel low, discouraged, and unsettled. I know now that these times will pass. They always do. I cry when I need to cry. I laugh when I need to laugh. Each day I engage in my spiritual practices such as Lectio Divina bible reading and Christian mindfulness meditation. From time to time, I write my prayers in a journal as I know this helps, especially if I can't sleep. I reflect on the things I feel most grateful for, and those that have been less uplifting. I remind myself of the sense I have of being loved. I so value the mutually healing interactions with the people who matter to me. I value my friendships and love the regular contact with my sons, my siblings, and my extended family both here in Aotearoa and overseas. I value my local church community and the prayer group that, until lockdown, met each month at my prophetic friend Bev's home in Auckland.

There is probably so much more of the detail of my life I could include. Increasingly, I am finding that my voice is working better than it has done since the tardive dystonia limited my ability for conversation 20 years ago. A major turning point occurred in 2013, on the trip to Lindisfarne with a friend. The church there has a reputation for maintaining 900 years of unbroken prayer, and my friend wrote a note to ask the prayer team to include healing of my voice in their prayers. The next day I suddenly noticed I was speaking with ease, and this remarkable relief lasted until I returned to New Zealand several weeks later. Strangely, the initial healing was temporary, but there has been a steady improvement since then. In a literal way, I am finding my voice.

Recently, I called in to say hello to the people at Buchanan Rehab Centre as I sometimes do when I am in the area. I was greeted with many hugs, which I returned with affection. It always feels like visiting family or whanau. I was delighted to hear that the staff were still using the language of 'victorious cycles' and seeing crises as opportunities for building more resilience. I was encouraged to know that the electronic recording categories that we developed were still in place (now 15 or more years later) and that 'being with' was still valued as a central focus of care. Indeed, the clinical director at the time was ensuring that regular audits were carried out to support this practice, together with all the other elements of the 'Re-covery Model'. As far as I know, they are still embedded in the system and the ethos of the service. 'Building a Bridge of Trust' was mentioned as a major component of practice.

I'm proud to say that my original research (Randal et al., 2003) was included in a meta-analysis of studies published over the past 25 years that investigated psychotherapy for people with so-called treatment resistance (Polese, Fornaro, Palermo, De Luca, & De Bartolomeis, 2019). Not many people in the world have attempted to do research of this sort, let alone found statistically significant positive outcomes. Inclusion of my work in this meta-analysis feels personally and professionally validating.

Having retired from my clinical role, in 2015, I spent nine precious months living in England, close to my mother during her final days. I treasure every minute of the time we had together. Images of the whole family reuniting around her bedside and celebrating her life with her in our midst remain as a jewel in my memory. But an unexpected gift was meeting the man in whose house I was lodging. I'm not sure if it was love at first sight exactly, but our lodger/landlord relationship gradually blossomed into a sweet friendship.

I was surprised by how much we enjoyed one another's company, doing the simple things of life together – shopping and cooking, sharing a meal and a glass of wine, walking and talking, going to movies or out dancing and dining, and more intimate things. Every minute was great fun. When it was time for me to return to New Zealand, he came with me for three months to be my lodger, reversing the roles until the time came for him to leave.

Over the past five years, apart from brief holidays together in America, England, and New Zealand, we mainly communicated by email. We have lots in common despite many differences in our backgrounds. Both of us were bruised by being left by our spouses over a decade before we met. We each have three sons of similar ages. We are sharing our faith journeys albeit from different perspectives – reading and reflecting together from the same books and blog sites. Having established lives 12,000 miles apart has not made it easy. There have been times of radio silence when each of us has been trying to figure out how to proceed. But it feels as if we are at a new chapter in our story, or maybe beginning a new book. Being in solitary confinement on opposite sides of the planet because of the pandemic brought us even closer together. Frequent Skype calls are adding to our sense of connectedness. Maybe once the world has found a new way forward following the Corona virus crisis, we will find a new way forward too. Whatever happens, I will always be grateful for the happiness our friendship has brought.

I have enjoyed writing this book and I will miss it now that it is finished. Life has been good to me and I trust that the best is yet to come.

JOSEPHINE'S STORY 1998
TO PRESENT DAY (AGES 44–65)

27

BECOMING A PSYCHIATRIST

A Pathway of Impossible Jobs

In which Josephine outlines her path towards finding a place to contribute within institutional psychiatry.

I had negotiated the exam process. I could 'psychiatrise' anyone; assess them, develop a treatment plan and put it into practice. I had confidence in my ability to analyse the academic literature. I had arrived. Even as I felt the achievement, I had a nagging sense of a hollowness.

Child psychiatry was the area I chose to work in. Part of the attraction was a small but cohesive and supportive group of child psychiatrists in Auckland. Child psychiatry focused much more on psychological and holistic approaches with involvement of family and systems, and much less use of medication than adult psychiatry.

My first job as a psychiatrist was half-time in the acute inpatient unit where I am working now. Despite all the knowledge and skills I had acquired, I found working in the inpatient unit just too hard. The young people were the most complex and risky patients who could not be managed in the community. Families would often arrive with a sense of relief that now they would finally get what their child needed. We so often disappointed them. Young people just wanted to leave. Nursing staff found it very frustrating to be trying to give care to these reluctant young people who they knew would be better off out of hospital. I felt I couldn't please anybody.

In the other half of my week, I had another flirtation with an academic career, setting up a postgraduate course in child and adolescent mental health for clinicians with adult qualifications. The first year was a bit of a whirlwind. Staying a step ahead of the course as it ran was a struggle but I managed it – just. Despite, and perhaps partly because of, running on the edge of chaos, there was a vibrant energy to the course and I loved meeting the students. They were the clinicians who had stepped into the gap to develop child and adolescent mental health services. How they managed the work involved in the course on top of their full-time jobs is still a mystery to me. The course is still running and has developed greatly in the intervening decades.

DOI: 10.4324/9781003153788-37

In order to pay the mortgage for the house we had bought that we could not afford, I opened a private practice on Thursday evenings and Saturday mornings. Working with the private patients who were choosing and paying to see me was interesting, and mostly I felt I could offer something helpful. But the combination was all tiring.

In January 1999, I was sitting having my breakfast, about to go back to work following my summer holiday. Rather than my usual sense of anticipation, curiosity, and interest, I felt a heaviness. Something needed to change. A friend had repeatedly approached me to work in a child and adolescent community service she was setting up in Northland. It would pay enough to enable me to give up the inpatient work and the private practice. It was an impossible job, providing cover in two days a week for a large semi-rural area with about 150,000 people and little chance of employing qualified staff. Other friends counselled me against it, but though the Northland job might be impossible, at least it was a different impossible. As I had from my childhood I did not entertain the possibility that I would not be able to manage.

After the first couple of months, I thought I had made a dreadful mistake. So much was needed but I and the woman who was setting up the team were the only ones with specific training and skills in child psychiatry assessment and treatment. The other team members were committed and energetic. Many had worked in adult mental health. What they lacked in specific child and adolescent mental health skills they made up in life experience, commitment, flexibility, local knowledge, and understanding of the worlds people lived in. We had to find a way of harnessing all this to enrich the lives of the children, young people, and families who came to us.

We developed a system where two clinicians met with the young person and family, in their home if possible, and asked them about their worries, their hopes, their experiences, and their relationships. It might take two hours or more. Often significant change would happen as a result of this initial conversation. The clinicians would bring a summary of what they had learnt to our team review meeting. We would then think together about what we could offer, making use of other services – structured questionnaires and pieces of manualised therapy drawn from Cognitive Behavioural Therapy (CBT) and Dialectical Behaviour Therapy (DBT). The team members engaged wholeheartedly in supporting parents, young people, and schools by listening and encouraging all to participate in building lives worth living for the young people. When my input was needed, I would join the clinician with the young person and family working within the relationship they had built. Over time, the staff increased their DBT and CBT skills, similar to the strategies Patte taught.

We developed a group approach to teaching DBT skills. We worked with a number of young people who were lurching from crisis to crisis. They described feeling fine in a session with a therapist but, when they walked out the door, they felt they still had nothing to help them. I had been to a seminar on DBT and as I listened to this description, I thought of DBT skills as something to take away from a session. We began with a group for staff and one young person. When I went on leave, a young nurse took over the group and, with the support of clinicians doing similar interventions in other services, developed handouts and a guide for running a DBT-like group in our service. Teaching DBT skills to troubled young people became an effective way our staff could engage, without getting caught up in the emotional turmoil.

Another impossible job which needed to be filled came up. This was as a child psychiatrist in a community service in Auckland, which had not had a permanent, child psychiatrist working there for more than a decade. There had been a series of foreign locums, of variable quality. It had been an exciting challenge setting up the university course, but my passion lay in pushing the boundaries of what we were offering people, rather than teaching the standard wisdom. I was also aware that doing what was needed to work at the top of my game in three careers – teacher, researcher, and clinician – seemed too hard.

There was limited satisfaction in this new clinical role. Being stretched so thinly, it was difficult to build good working relationships with staff, let alone young people and families. This was not helped by the challenges they had experienced in engaging with a succession of locum psychiatrists. Some young people had had new treatment plans with each new psychiatrist. When I could see what I thought was a better plan, I had to weigh up the possible benefits of my revised plan against the unsettling experience for them of proposing yet another change.

After four or five years there, other psychiatrists were coming on stream and so the need for my work there became less acute. Over this time, I had been developing my ideas on how I wanted to work more collaboratively. Engaging in private practice for some days of the week seemed like an opportunity for more freedom from institutional requirements and to continue to develop my own path.

However, I found yet another impossible job. The acute child and adolescent inpatient unit I had worked in six years before was in crisis. There were dire shortages of both nurses and psychiatrists. It was a critical gap which desperately needed filling. Taking on this job would be completely different from what I had planned. In comparison to private practice, acute inpatient care was a much more complex testing ground for working collaboratively. Applying these principles in the context of providing compulsory care for people with high levels of risk and psychosis would teach me more. There was also a sense of unfinished business as I had found work in the inpatient unit so difficult to manage six years before. The possibility that I could find it similarly overwhelming at this time was not something I allowed to enter my mind.

Even with my additional clinical experience, I still found the acute inpatient work very hard. The challenges seemed insurmountable. The physical environment was not nurturing, tucked into a basement with minimal outside area. We had over 20 referrers covering the top half of the North Island with many more than 20 different ideas of what they hoped for from us. We served an age range from birth to 18. Despite all this, over about five years, we were able to build a positive work environment which attracts good staff.

Critical to the forward movements we made was a solid leadership group. This was not an institutional structure but an informal group made up of like-minded senior nurses, psychiatrists, and a manager. We used consensus decision-making. If someone disagreed with an idea the rest supported, we didn't focus on bringing them around to our way of thinking. We had such respect for each other that we knew that we would all gain from listening and fully understanding why they were seeing the situation differently. We learnt to take any new idea to the 'old guard' – group members who had been around in the unit longest – to actively seek their knowledge of potential pitfalls in the early stages of adopting an idea. Their cautions felt like helpful information. Otherwise, there was a risk they might appear to be undermining attempts at innovation with prophecies of doom and gloom.

I am still working there after 17 years.

28

MY ALTERNATIVE TRAINING
Pathway to Becoming the Psychiatrist I Want to Be

> In which Josephine describes some of the rich experiences which have enabled her to find a way to contribute to shifting the culture of psychiatry.

Learning from Patte

Patte was pregnant with her youngest child when I met her in my first year of training. Her creative energy, alternative ideas, and passion for her work attracted my attention. It became clear to me that she thought things through and worked with ideas with a level of sophistication I didn't often come across. When she alluded to having had an experience of psychosis, I could not put this together with the articulate, highly intelligent and interpersonally attuned young woman before me. She seemed a testament to the idea of an experience of psychosis as an opportunity. But how was I to process all of this in the context of the pathologising psychiatric discourse I was trying to become an expert in?

The clinical work Patte did fascinated and perplexed me. I saw her approach a young person and invite them to come and talk with her. Her body language and tone inferred one person asking another a favour. The expert role I was aiming to perfect, involved exuding the confidence that I was well equipped to offer the person something important and valuable for their lives. This would leave them in no doubt that it would serve them to accede to my polite and respectful direction. I am glad I have these skills and can bring them out when useful, but I have had to do considerable unlearning of this approach and find other ways.

What Patte was doing was 'wrong' in several ways, according to what I was being taught. As she has described, we were taught that psychotherapy was 'contra-indicated' for people with psychosis. The risk of making people with susceptibility to psychosis worse was demonstrated by the anecdote I described in the residential psychotherapy programme (Chapter 15). I also saw this happen in Odyssey House, the residential substance-dependence treatment programme. Some of the people came from the adult mental health

DOI: 10.4324/9781003153788-38

unit, where they had seemed fine, but they would decompensate into acute psychotic states after only a few days. Both these programmes were quite confronting with a high level of interpersonal contact. This atmosphere was not therapeutic for people at risk for psychosis. What Patte was doing was finding a way to do therapy which was safe for people, even when they were actively experiencing psychosis.

When I read Patte's account of the work she did in her research, the care she took is so clear. At the time I did not know what to make of it. She was working from her own creativity and intuition, rather than following a manualised, evidence-based treatment. It was very different from what I was being taught. Whenever I heard her talk about her work, it tapped into my discomfort that we were offering people so little. Knowing how to be helpful to people in psychotic states felt challenging to me. It seemed that Patte's own experience of psychosis contributed – but it was more than this.

When Patte rang me to tell me she was not being reappointed to the training scheme, I was dumbfounded and flooded with feelings. Apart from feeling for her my selfish response was fear. If they were doing this to her, what would they do to me if they found out about the ambivalence I had, regarding our psychiatric training? I did not, at the time have the insight to realise I was quite safe in working so hard to be a more ordinary rat. But it shattered my world view. Had those people, who were supposed to be providing leadership in the training programme and psychiatry in Auckland, lost their way? What was I doing, trying to make myself into a psychiatrist?

Not for a moment did I think it was a good decision that Patte should not be a psychiatrist. My sister remembers my talking to her about wanting to advocate for Patte in some way but not feeling able to. Her work and ideas were not in line with what we were being taught but I knew that the people we were trying to serve needed something different. My intuitive sense was that what had happened to Patte was another example where established institutional ideas were being held onto at the expense of the openness that is required for forward movement.

Looking back now, I know the people who were on the training committee were thoughtful people who volunteered to serve on it out of a commitment to psychiatry – to making things better. At the heart of their concern was protecting the vulnerable people who seek support and care from psychiatrists. Managing a system to train psychiatrists to hold the institutional power vested in us is a complex task. There was limited understanding at the time of the value of lived experience, and how to use it. Prior to our study, psychotic illness in doctors was barely acknowledged in the literature. Times are changing and we are hoping that this book will contribute to that change.

Patte and I enjoyed rich and varied companionship. We rattled around with our preschoolers and walked and talked with and without our children and dogs. We talked about work, children, family, friends, philosophical ideas – everything and anything. At times when I felt I might have done something unwise at work, she always felt the safest person to have a first discussion with. Despite the different ways we approached our work, I never felt judged or 'less than' in our conversations. They almost always led to an opening in my thinking, to different possibilities, and often ideas about something constructive I could do.

As I continued my psychiatry apprenticeship, polishing my ability to jump through the right hoops and identifying increasingly strongly with the dominant psychiatry model, she kept me in touch with other developments. These included the hearing voices network, the value of experience-based expertise, the Recovery Movement, and later the Open Dialogue approach. There was an aspect of discomfort to all this. It would have been much more straightforward to move into the role of psychiatrist, without taking account of other ways of understanding what we were doing. Probably what I found most painful was Patricia Deegan's describing mental health services as 'spirit breaking' (Deegan, 1990). I could see the truth in that.

Patte's losing her voice unsettled me. It was so difficult for her to talk that, when on phone calls, I would talk in a way that meant she could participate with as few words as possible. Seeing something so debilitating, and apparently permanent, happening to someone close to me was much more confronting than the research knowledge I had about the range of side effects. It conflicted with my wanting to feel I was doing something good for people. And yet, had I been her psychiatrist, I may well have advocated long-term risperidone for Patte. I was prescribing it and other similar medications for people. I still am.

The excitement about the second-generation 'antipsychotics', the first of which was risperidone, had infected me too. They weren't supposed to cause all the problems we had with the old ones. It is only while writing this book that I learned about the money that was paid by drug companies to the academic psychiatrists who publicised risperidone. The slow realisation that risperidone was actually very little different from the older medications was hard to process.

Patte's talk about spiritual emergency seemed to provide a possibility for an alternative to the understanding of psychosis as a chronic, disabling condition. In looking for spiritual emergencies as an alternative to psychotic illness, I had conceptualised a crisis which would not need medication. Rather, it would need a specific intervention for resolving the spiritual emergency. There were many people I met who seemed to be overwhelmed with spiritual and existential issues in the context of psychosis, but I could not see what to do. We did not seem to be able to make progress without antipsychotic medication. Working on the book, I have come to realise that it is not a matter of *either* a spiritual emergency *or* psychosis, but *both*. What *is* important is listening to the detail and the meaning in people's experience. Patte describes resolving her spiritual emergence as being a process of evolution over years, including a number of extreme experiences. If we think about spirituality as about finding meaning in life, and psychosis as a crisis of meaning-making, then there may be a spiritual element to any psychosis.

Even just holding in mind the contradictions between my view and Patte's perspectives and experience supported me to hold the paradigm of psychiatry I worked in more lightly. The everyday influence on my clinical work would be in a combination of 'being with' and listening carefully for what had meaning for the person. It doesn't sound like much when I put it like that, but when I manage to do it, it makes a difference. As we have worked together on this book, describing her approach and the tools she has developed, my work has been reinvigorated.

There have been many times when I have been in a situation where I have experienced pressure from the dominant model, or other clinicians, or services to enforce compulsory care in a way which has a risk of being spirit-breaking. It would save me considerable worry and potential conflict to go along with the dominant forces. But thinking *What would Patte say?* helps me focus on holding the perspective of the person at risk in the forefront of my mind.

A laminated illustration of the Bridge of Trust was the first of Patte's tools I used. When people appeared to be struggling to engage, I often used to ask them directly how easy it was to feel as if we were there to help, or if they were wondering if we might do them harm. The Bridge of Trust diagram helped this process. It was easier for both of us to be looking at a diagram which softened the intensity of the one-on-one interaction. The cards about *When I am at my best* would be the other thing I have used the most.

There are some young people for whom it seems much easier to do practical tasks than answer questions. Most of us ask and respond to the question, 'How are you?' many times a day. But it is not a straightforward question. An answer is often not wanted, and if it is, the nature of the socially appropriate answer varies with the context. This complexity and ambiguity are such a contrast to being asked to find the right place for the cursor on the feelometer. This is particularly relevant for a young person in an extreme state, in a social context they have not had a chance to work out yet, with people they don't know.

Similarly, choosing cards from a set laid out on a table is an easier task than generating contributions to a conversation.

In the acute context, I do not have the opportunity to work through the whole 'Re-covery' plan, but using tools helps my conversations. Young people who are struggling to engage in talking about their experiences seem to be much happier choosing cards from a set laid out on a table than feeling pressure to generate answers to questions. Choosing cards from *When I am at my best* can be a welcome, forward looking, optimistic focus. Often the young person and I will come up with some steps to take as a result of even one or two brief conversations. Not everyone likes this approach. Having all the tools Patte has developed over the years brought together and presented in 'The Gift Box', which Patte describes in Chapter 30, works well for me.

It looks inviting and always attracts interest. Some young people who avoid conversations seem happy to come and talk with me when we are using these tools in 'The Gift Box'. Sometimes I don't even open it, because we get engaged in something else the young person wants to talk about.

Learning from People's Lived Experience

This began with the laborious histories I took as a medical student and has continued through my career. Opportunities can be surprisingly limited. For much of my career I have gone to work each day knowing that there is more work to complete than I can reasonably do justice to. It has been hard to *be with* people in a way that enabled me to hear their experience, when I am feeling under pressure to assess for diagnosis, make decisions about recommendations for treatment, and meanwhile take responsibility for people's safety.

In any personal contact, we hear only a fraction of the other's experience. A couple of examples remind me of how we often have no idea about extreme experiences people are having. One was a young man with a psychotic illness who did not want to sit and talk. He looked preoccupied and restless, but there was nothing else in the way he appeared that seemed out of the ordinary. As I accompanied him in pacing around the corridors, he told me how he had to hold back a tidal wave or we would all be engulfed. He spoke of his nana, his mum, and other members of his family. He seemed tormented by the responsibility and the worry that he would be unable to prevent their deaths.

Another was a quiet, apparently self-contained, neatly presented young woman who seemed to be finding it hard to answer my questions. Attending carefully to the detail of her experience, I came to some understanding of why this was. She was working so hard to be perfect for everyone and applying such harsh critical evaluation to anything she might say that it was almost impossible for her to say anything. She was so afraid she would not get the description of her feelings right and would feel so bad about falling short. The pressure she put on herself to please and meet expectations was such that she would not decline my request to meet. But the conversation was torture. I could easily not have known.

Reading books, watching documentaries, and hearing conference presentations have also added richness to my understanding of what people might experience. Some comments I heard at a conference on an alternative nursing model, where half the participants were consumers, continue to guide me. A man stood up and described the assault to personal integrity and autonomy involved in being injected with medication against his will. Being involved in this process has never been the same for me since.

Qualitative research, interviewing a small number of people, and studying the transcripts in great detail gave me a formal opportunity to immerse myself in people's lived experience. Though I let go the idea of an academic career,

I retained a commitment to research. Choosing impossible jobs no one else wanted gave me some negotiating leverage. Dedicated research time was always a bottom line for me. But most of the research and writing I have done has been in my own time. I call it my hobby.

My first qualitative research project involved interviewing women who had killed their children. The women's experiences, from their extreme states leading to killing their much-loved child(ren), through to the process of finding a way to live with having done this, were heart rending accounts of suffering and courage. They told me about being trapped in a delusional world where they believed their children were at risk of such suffering that death was the only potential release. Some had attempted joint suicide and spoke of the layers and layers of grief and other emotions around rebuilding a life after finding that their baby was dead but they were not. They spoke of being cut off from contact with children, even their own surviving children and other relatives. They were seen as a potential danger, when the only danger they had been to any child was in the specific context of the delusional distortions they experienced while in an extreme state.

Having three young children myself when I was doing these interviews, I identified deeply with the anguish they described. I hope the papers we wrote have been useful to the international clinical and academic community. As with the challenge of writing up the study about doctors, it was hard to get across in academic papers the depth and richness that was added to my understanding of what people can go through. At the time it had felt peripheral to child psychiatry but now that we have opened mother-baby beds in the Child and Family Unit, it is extremely relevant to my clinical work. Decades later, the papers we wrote are still being cited (Stanton & Simpson, 2001, 2002, 2006; Stanton, Simpson, & Wouldes, 2000).

Interviewing the participants of our doctor-patient study taught me about experiencing extreme states as well as about myself, both as a doctor and as a person. Accounts of suffering I heard from people I connected with still resonate with me. Several people talked about continuing to function with dogged and heroic disregard for their own vulnerability. One person talked about how suicide had seemed like a rational choice in the context of the intense, sustained suffering of depression. Several described longing for kindness and responsiveness from clinicians. Some described the crucial difference it had made when they had an experience of clinicians who were able to connect with them as a person.

Accounts of how their experiences had contributed to the quality of what they offered their patients also stimulated my own reflections and awareness about what I am offering. Most of the doctor-patients, and some of the treating psychiatrists, talked about how valuable their own illness experiences had been in improving what they offered patients as doctors. But the added wisdom from their own lived experience remained hidden. There was nowhere to share it.

Writing this feels like a struggle, to summarise so much learning over years in a few paragraphs. It takes me back to all the work Patte and I did, trying to get so much across in academic articles. This process went on for over a decade. Working together was easier when we lived in the same city. Once Patte moved to a town 140 km away, we sometimes met half way between our homes. One day we met in Pokeno. The café there was humming – not a quiet, reflective spot. We found a place on the side of the road under a tree and spent the day sitting on plastic chairs, working through our second paper on the psychiatrist-doctor-patient interaction. There was so much more we wanted to say. This struggle to find a way of communicating the richness of our learning led to this book.

Learning from Johnella Bird

Having had the opportunity to travel the world and learn from some of the most widely acclaimed clinicians, I found inspiration on my doorstep. Johnella Bird had begun her career as a child psychotherapist and worked extensively in narrative and family therapy towards developing her own therapeutic approach. I picked up one of her books at a Michael White workshop, which sparked my interest.

In the first workshop of hers I attended, there were about a dozen of us from a broad range of work contexts, mostly quite different from mine. Johnella is a tall athletic looking woman with a cloud of blond curly hair. She has an alert presence in the room, offering an intensely focused nurturing attention. She began the workshop by talking about her work in a way I felt drawn to but found puzzling at the same time.

Demonstrations of her work I found arresting. When a course member brought up a clinical challenge, she would ask them to take up the role of the person they were working with, while she took the role of the therapist. Nothing had prepared me for her method. In taking notes, I found that the only useful thing to do was write her questions verbatim. She shifted the usual use of language, which I would immediately forget if I didn't write it down. It sounded quite ordinary as I listened to it, but it wasn't.

Even in my first, inept efforts to use what I was learning to shift my work, I noticed a difference. It became possible to find ways through challenging conversations with a lightness and optimism that was new. My medical training had been about asking people questions to identify deficit, to get information into my head, so that I could figure out what was wrong and make a plan for how to fix it. This was also a pattern in individual psychotherapy assessment and family therapy. In the latter part of my training, there was growing interest in strengths, but this was often as a discrete area of inquiry, as in 'add strengths and stir'.

In Johnella's approach, the person's resources are central. The purpose of a question was not to get information into my head, but for the person to experience a shift, becoming more consciously aware of their own resources. Resources include values, hopes, intentions, things they are doing, tenacity they show, love they feel, and much more. An example I come across often is a family meeting where a parent is lecturing a child who is looking morose and disengaged. You don't have to be a very clever clinician to identify the fault in this sort of conversation. In Johnella's approach, I might ask the parent what they were hoping their child would take from what they were saying – that is, identify their intention.

One morning in Northland, when I was looking at the list of people I was going to see that day, I saw there was a family from a remote area with whom we had struggled to engage. They had refused several offers of regular appointments but been squeezed in because the children were on the verge of being expelled from school.

It was hard to feel enthusiasm for doing assessments on two children with complicated histories, in a time slot which was not enough for one. The school probably would not even be interested in all the information I would pull together into a letter. Other families I was supposed to see that day would also end up getting a bit less.

But it didn't have to be like that. I wasn't an expert on their lives. I wouldn't have known how to manage these challenging children with the level of adversity this mother negotiated. She was making very different choices in raising her children from those I would have made, but she was doing it. She loved them, and they felt loved and belonging in their community. They didn't need a psychiatric expert. Identifying psychiatric disorders wouldn't help. She had no interest in the sort of thinking or the interventions we offered. The school might not be particularly interested either.

But I did have something to offer. I structured a conversation focused on getting the kids' mother to talk about how she had decided to make the choices she had made, and how well they were working for the family. As I got them all to talk about how they wanted to be at school – times when things worked for them, what was bothering the school, and what would make a difference – I started engaging in the conversation; it was a fascinating journey of joint discovery. All sorts of things came up which I would never have thought about.

The letter to the school was a summary of stories they were sharing, and observations I made about their taking up agency in their lives. I never found out exactly how they negotiated the immediate crisis, but the children stayed in school and did end up engaging in the service in a more regular way later. The rest of the families I saw that day got an energised, rather than a depleted, psychiatrist to meet with them. It might have made a contribution to their lives. It was a point of radical change to mine.

Letting go of trying to be the expert on other people's lives was a weight off my shoulders. My psychiatric expertise was always available, but I was also developing expertise in supporting conversations which brought people's resources into their conscious awareness. This meant they were accessible to them to use to improve their lives. If I heard someone had made what I thought was a poor decision, I could ask, 'How did you decide to do that?' The focus of the question was not identifying deficits, but understanding and identifying values or intentions. If I thought someone had done something rather unwise, I could ask, 'How well did that work for you?' They were usually able to tell me something much more useful about the limitations of their choice than I had thought of.

An example of this was of a woman who came in to an outpatient appointment with her preadolescent child. As is common in child psychiatry, the child had no interest in being there and wanted to leave. She suggested the child go to a nearby shop to buy something to eat and come back. As they discussed how much was OK to spend and what to do with the change, I noticed myself judging her, thinking she seemed unable to set a boundary. Instead of deciding this was an area I needed to teach her something about, I asked her how she had made the decision to do what she did. As she talked about her thinking process, I realised how sensitively and thoughtfully she was negotiating a challenging situation with a mildly autistic child who was struggling with anxiety, hating being told what to do and, at the same time, needing guidance. She could reflect on how well the strategies she used worked or didn't work in different situations. At the end of the conversation, I had developed profound respect for her parenting. This gave us a chance to work usefully together. It also took me off the hook from having to come up with the solutions.

As I built more facility in using Johnella's ideas, I found it increased the joy and decreased the burden I experienced in my clinical work. I wanted to share it. This resulted in a rude shock in a very public forum when I naively attempted to share my ideas about talking with children and families about Attention Deficit Hyperactivity Disorder (ADHD).

Children and families seemed to engage more readily with the idea of ADHD as a personal style rather than something wrong with them. This is internally inconsistent given what ADHD stands for, Attention Deficit Hyperactivity Disorder, but it seemed to work. I talked about an ADHD style, with an increased level of impulsivity, increased level of activity and decreased ability to keep attention narrowly focused. This style is not helpful in the classroom. But in other contexts, such as for a soldier, a farmer or a harbour master, it could be helpful to be perpetually on the go, have a roving, rather than narrowly focused attention and be able to react quickly without too much deliberating. ADHD style people can be fun to be with. My sense was that families, children, and young people found this helpful and were happy to look at strategies and explore medication to help in situations like the classroom, long car journeys, or visits to certain relatives.

Thinking that other child psychiatrists might also find this approach helpful, I wrote a letter describing it to the prestigious Journal of the American

Academy of Child and Adolescent Psychiatry. One night after getting out of the taxi from the airport as I was coming back from Northland, I saw the orange American Academy Journal in the mail on the table. Flicking through it, I felt quite excited to find my letter. But a hot flush of shame spread over me when I read a letter from two big international names in ADHD research, ripping my letter to shreds. This public vilification from such prestigious people for someone as insignificant as me seemed a lot of trouble to go to. Did defending the deficit-focused model mean more to them than the possibility of having more helpful conversations with families? I managed to pull myself together to write a response. This was again crushed by the big names. These have been my most requested publications (Stanton, 2003, 2005).

Applying and doing my best to spread these ideas and strategies to enable a shift away from a deficit focus has been my conscious contribution to shifting the paradigm in psychiatry. I did a number of presentations at my workplaces and at national and international conferences. A colleague and I developed a website, www.talkthatheals.org outlining practical strategies from Johnella's approach which can be picked up by any clinician. In writing this book, we have extended the website to include Patte's work.

A randomised, controlled trial would have been the most effective way to make Johnella's work more available. It would have been possible, still is, but so much work. As with Patte's research, there would have been the research proposal to write, ethics approval to get, and funding to secure before I could begin. I would have had to develop a fidelity scale to be clear that the work the intervention clinicians were doing fitted her approach. Then I would have to engage clinicians, services, and managers in the training and use of the approach. Then we would need to identify and enrol participants in the study, analyse the data, and write it all up for publication. Controlled trials are vital to developing an evidence base but require so much resource to perform. It was beyond me. How many other ideas never reach clinicians who could use them to make a difference to people's lives because trials are not done?

Self-Determination Theory

A few years ago, I stumbled across Self-Determination Theory. It is a well-researched psychological theory that well-being and internal motivation are increased when people experience relatedness, autonomy, and competence. I was stunned. This encapsulated the essence of everything I had been working towards, with an evidence base. Ever since I began my training in psychiatry, I had felt mildly subversive with an intuitive sense that something else was needed. The Recovery Movement put much of that into words and then, when I found Johnella's work, I had a technology, a way of developing skills and tools to put it into practice. But I had always been aware that my way of working was consistently counter-cultural. Here, in Self-Determination Theory, were decades of a research tradition supporting everything I believed in and aspired to practise. Research we have done seeking young people's experiences of being in the unit supports the importance of addressing these needs (Stanton, Thomas, Jarbin, & Mackay, 2020).

Learning from Sports Coaches

The coaches of my daughters' netball in primary school had a wealth of knowledge about how to play netball, but they did almost no telling. They were always warm and encouraging. At training they used exercises for the kids to build skills. During the matches, the only advice they gave was for the children to 'make space' and 'look down', towards their goal. This seemed odd to me. Even with my very limited netball skills, I could often see what I thought the kids should be doing. Some parents with a bit more confidence did advise their kids from the sideline. It was obvious that it resulted in the kids playing worse. It was a powerful lesson in the importance of finding other ways of enabling people to develop their skills other than telling.

Through my son's sailing and windsurfing, I have been able to observe Grant Beck who has coached a number of Olympic gold medallists. His sons were part of the same club. Like the netball coaches he was endlessly warm, validating, and positive. The focus was on discovery rather than telling. He would ask the kids what they had done to go faster and created opportunities for them to watch and learn from each other. Using similar methods, he has enabled the Olympic champions to learn more about windsurfing than he ever knew and reach a standard he never achieved himself.

Grant had less expertise in the competitive sport than some of the people he was coaching. But he was expert in supporting a process to bring out the best in them. This resonated with Johnella's work. She is an expert, but not in living people's lives, or what they should do. She is an expert in managing a conversation in the therapeutic relationship to bring forward the best in the person seeking her help. When I can remember that I have less expertise in living people's lives than they do, and refrain from telling, keeping the focus on bringing out their resources, I notice I am at my most useful for people.

Learning from Eckhart Tolle

Along with all the other exploring I have done, I have also always looked around a range of spiritual traditions. The writings of Eckhart Tolle have been especially helpful. They enable me to be present in the now, refocus, and let go in a way which can transform my experience of life and work. His messages are found in many places. My natural bent is to engage with intensity, taking on challenges with positive energy. This approach often serves me well, but I can also waste energy in frustration with what I cannot change. Where I work in an inpatient unit, this opportunity is frequently available. Young people often enter inpatient units in crisis. Their families and referrers

205

have hopes and expectations we cannot possibly meet. Too often they fail to see the work we do and highlight our shortcomings energetically. Arguing back is less than helpful. Just as we are, they are doing their best in challenging circumstances. Eckhart Tolle's writings have supported me to surrender to what I cannot change and even experience joy. Focusing on presence, and stilling the mind, is invaluable in clinical work.

29

AGAINST ALL ODDS
Maintaining My Personal and Professional Identity

In which Josephine reflects on what she contributes.

Sometimes I wonder if I would have taken a different path if I had known at 22 what I know now, but I love my work. Becoming a psychiatrist, developing expertise in this particular way of understanding and engaging with people, has taken significant effort. I have always worked within institutions where this approach is entrenched. The social construction of the role of medical specialists in our society supports a pathologising discourse. Assessment, provision of solutions, and being told what to do from an expert position is what people expect from us. My aim is to bring what I offer as a psychiatrist, together with other possibilities in a process of discovery.

This is what I aspire to. Particularly when tired and stressed, I notice myself taking up the expert position, pathologising, and telling. This is like the registrars who came to Patte's teaching and felt inspired by it to practise differently, but found they couldn't. Like the frogs in slowly heating water, we have all been acclimatised to the predominant culture, not by our choice, mostly without even noticing.

Working with registrars reminds me how far I have shifted. Recently, I was with a registrar reviewing a young person who had just arrived at the unit. The focus at this time is on what the young person (and family if they are there) wants to get out of the admission and how we support them with their safety over the next day or so. The registrar asked the young person what they understood the rationale for the admission to be. The young person described their understanding of what clinicians were thinking, and the conversation moved into deficit and disorders. Stepping in, I asked the young person what they personally wanted from the admission. The conversation became much lighter and forward-focused. The subtlety in the difference between the two questions belies its power. Focusing on what the young person and family think, rather than on the expertise of professionals, is surprisingly countercultural.

Supervising registrars is a particular challenge and opportunity. They are working hard to master the deficit-focused, expert-based dominant models of

DOI: 10.4324/9781003153788-39

psychiatry and psychotherapy. I want to help them with that, and I also want them to have an opportunity, at the very least, to realise there are other possibilities. Joint clinical practice is particularly hard. A focus I am developing on joint discovery is so different from what they need to learn to pass their exams or the telling and reassuring which come so easily to all of us. Stepping in, as described above, has the risk of undermining their clinical practice. They will learn and develop as clinicians best in a context where they feel supported and validated.

Working in a unit where I have been able to join with like-minded clinicians to build a different sort of culture is such a privilege. Recently, I was with a suicidal young person and their family. We weren't managing to engage the young person in working with us and their suicidal feelings were becoming an increasing focus. My anxiety was rising and I found myself wanting to take control and lock the young person up for their own safety. However, I also knew this had a risk of creating a vicious cycle of our taking control, the young person becoming increasingly resentful, and our ability to work together being even further undermined, thus increasing the risk. Few clinicians in that situation have the luxury I had of being able to leave the room and check out my concerns with the nurses. Together we made a plan to support the young person without transferring them from the open ward to the locked area. We moved out of battle mode and over a couple of days things moved forward. Being part of creating and supporting the culture in the unit feels deeply satisfying.

Like most of us, I do my best. I get it wrong sometimes, but I hope I am contributing in my small way to the changes that mean so much to me. Sometimes I get affirmation of this, often in surprising ways. Long before electric scooters were popular, I began riding a push scooter to work. A number of people seem to get a buzz about seeing an old lady scooting herself along. As I crossed Ponsonby Road one morning, a man sitting at a café gave me the thumbs up and said, 'You are my inspiration'. It made my day.

PATTE'S STORY

30

CREATIVE ENERGY AND 'THE GIFT BOX'

In which Patte packages up her life's work into 'The Gift Box'
with promising developments and unlimited possibilities.

A cold, windy day in Auckland, in 2013. The sky is that dull grey colour that makes everything look faded and worn out. At least it's not raining, so my autumn work clothes are dry on the outside and I'm only a bit sweaty from rushing to get there on time. In my eco-friendly tote bag are all the bits and pieces that make up my 'Re-covery Model' resource kit – the box of colour-coded cards, the feelometer, the maps, and diagrams. Josephine and I have been meeting for weeks now, sitting together on an uncomfortable couch in the hospital photographer's office, making a teaching video of a role play to showcase my invention. Hilariously, Josephine has been acting the part of a 17 year old. She knows adolescents inside out. She becomes Annabel the moment the camera is turned on.

'Hello Annabel', I say. 'How has your week been? Today we'll be having a look at everything we've learned in the past twelve sessions. Where would you put yourself on the feelometer right now?'

Annabel takes the feelometer from me and places the cursor on 70. She pauses for a moment, looking into her lap, where she has balanced her completed 'Re-covery' workbook on her knees.

'It's been good'. She pauses again, maintaining the suspense. 'I saw my Mum'.

She eyes me silently, waiting for a response. I smile with genuine pleasure. This is a creative reconstruction of a young woman's life, only loosely based on reality, but I can feel the joy behind the acting. Josephine knows what it's like to make breakthroughs with young people who have struggled with hearing voices and self-harm.

'Oh wow! That's wonderful! Last week it seemed like an impossible task. Sounds like you're making real steps towards that victorious cycle you've been hoping for. I was at about 60 on the feelometer

DOI: 10.4324/9781003153788-41

when I got here – didn't sleep well, and it was hard to find a car park. Now I'm at 70 too, after hearing that news! Do you want to tell me how you did that?'

It's easy for me to be in the role, as I'm playing myself. We complete the session, I say goodbye to Josephine, and make a time to go back to see the hard-working photographer when he has had a chance to edit all those recorded hours down to a digestible length.

A couple of weeks later, I'm entering the city hospital on my way to sign off the video project. I've brought everything with me so that close up photographs can be taken for the finished product. As I run for the lift, I catch sight of a shiny poster inviting medical staff to attend an 'Innovation Workshop'. I've never heard of such a thing. The start time is exactly following the scheduled end of my meeting, and the room is just along the same corridor.

Heaving the straps of my tote bag over my shoulder, I wonder if my cards, feelometer, diagrams, and ideas would constitute an innovation. This thought carries me to that workshop and beyond.

Within a few days, I'm sitting in my office at Buchanan Rehabilitation Centre with a young man looking over my shoulder. He's the handsome pre-senter who so enthusiastically detailed the vision for advancing medical innov-ation with the help of government funding. I'm explaining how the 'Re-covery Model' works, tracing the spiral pathway as we re-cover patterns of resilience and vulnerability that have developed throughout our variably traumatic lives from conception until now, reframing crises as opportunities to turn vicious cycles into victorious cycle. I explain how all the resources fit together. He is a keen listener. He even has a go with the feelometer. He gets the concepts imme-diately, even though he has no clinical or mental health training.

'The only problem', he says with concern, 'is that all this stuff you've developed is not a thing. You can't market it if it's not a *thing*'.

My mind tumbles backwards through time, retrieving some words that had been lodged in my memory several years earlier:

'Compete in the marketplace.' Bev, a lively and intelligent eld-erly woman in my church with a reputation for giving accurate prophecy, had deposited this phrase in my surprised ears at choir practice one evening. These words had seemed so out of place. I was a clinician working in the public system. Competing in the marketplace was the last thing I imagined doing. How odd that these words are there to be recalled now. As I find myself thinking about making my invention marketable, inspiration comes to me in a flash.

'What if we put it all in a box?' I say. 'We could call it "The Gift Box".'

The young entrepreneur likes the idea. He leaves with a bounce in his step. The following weekend I enthusiastically tell a friend about 'The Gift Box'. She and her husband think it's a great idea too.

As if to reinforce the meant-to-be-ness of this as yet an unformed new *thing*, Bev turns up unexpectedly at a church meeting soon after, where this same friend and I happen to be sitting side by side. I have not seen Bev in the intervening years. She is carrying a small wooden box, and tells the gathered crowd:

> 'This is a very special box. It's a working man's box that belonged to my grandfather, and contained his protractor, but actually it was a precious *gift* that he left to the family. I feel I am to hand around this *gift box*, and anyone for whom this speaks or has meaning, please put up your hand and we will pray for you.'

I look at my friend in awe. She is nodding, laughing at the coincidence, urging me to raise my hand. I find myself surrounded by praying women, their warm hands placed on my arms and back, the top of my head. It feels like a done deal. I'm thrilled and amazed.

But even though quite a lot of trouble is taken to advance 'The Gift Box' proposal to the next level, the *thing* doesn't fly. Not just yet. Maybe it's not the right time.

Fast forward another few years, to 2017. Life is changing a lot for me. My work at Buchanan Centre has come to an end, but I have been encouraged along the way by various opportunities and invitations to present workshops as far afield as Liverpool and Sydney. 'The Gift Box' is taking shape in my mind, and now appears in the title of my presentations, even though nothing material has changed. Dozens of Australian workshop participants leave equipped with packets of cards, maps, and mini feelometers sticking out of their briefcases and handbags, fashioned by my generous hosts. I even hear about a 'Re-covery' group that has been going for ten years in an Australian town somewhere, instigated by a psychotherapist we trained at Buchanan, now long gone from Australia. Images of koalas, kangaroos, and those beautiful red and green parrots accompany my sense of achievement.

Bev's words continue to scaffold my motivation. 'Compete in the marketplace'. I wonder where this is heading and how far it will go.

In the middle of that winter, a younger woman friend contacts me to say she has just been in hospital and is recovering from another bout of psychosis. Can she come and see me? I invite her to stay for the weekend. We use the maps, diagrams, cards, workbooks, and feelometer to review the past months and years of her journey. The trust builds as I share more parts of my own story. Tears flow. Hugs abound. By the end of our intense 72 hours together, punctuated by healthy breakfasts and delicious vegetarian dinners, my friend has had an epiphany. Her *aha* moment comes when she puts together the chain reaction of how one event leads to another, and another – a vicious cycle of interactions that suddenly make more sense to her than ever before. We both feel uplifted by the renewed knowing that victorious cycles really happen, and that it means embracing our vulnerability and facing our pain.

Before she leaves, my friend presents me with a drawing she has made. It is a professionally crafted picture of 'The Gift Box', with accurate dimensions of shape and size. On the bottom of the page is a phone number and the name of a graphic designer in Rotorua. Little did I know that in her youth, this talented young woman had been a graphic designer herself, in partnership with this man to whom she is now referring me. She can see the potential for 'The Gift Box' idea to become a commercial entity. After her own experience with using the concepts and tools, she adds her creative energy to my dream.

But mundane life again overtakes me, and that valuable piece of paper sits unattended on my desk for another half year, until a meeting with the mother of a boy who has endured several hospital admissions for psychosis revives my impetus to move things forward again. I realise that it's about time I contacted Tony Hadlow, the name that my friend left for me to follow up, who turns out to have some wonderfully creative ideas about how to proceed with 'The Gift Box'.

Within months, there are 50 first-edition versions of 'The Gift Box' out in the world. Twenty are field-trialled in the Waikato, where I live, having moved from Auckland. Maybe by now some are gathering dust on shelves, admired but put aside for want of time or focused attention. Some, I know, have been put to good use over and over, and the recipients are themselves helping to co-facilitate 'Understanding Ourselves with "The Gift Box"' groups in the outer reaches of the district.

And then, mid-2019, a stranger taps on my car window: 'May I be so bold as to ask if you are single?'. In ordinary circumstances, I would have smiled warmly, thanked him for the courageous enquiry and told him I was unavailable. But something prompts me to invite him to tell me his story. He turns out to be a retired technical editor of instruction manuals. In retrospect, I doubt that there was anyone in New Zealand better suited to help me incorporate all the feedback I have received from the field trial. How do these things happen? Now, in 2020, we have produced 50 copies of the second edition of 'The Gift Box'.

In April 2020, in the middle of the Covid-19 lockdown, I was awarded a grant by an organisation named Ember Korowai Takitini to set up a hybrid project to research the implementation and effectiveness of the *thing* that is at last on the verge of competing in the marketplace. It is exciting, daunting, and uplifting all at the same time. I am encouraged to hear stories of young men in the local forensic unit choosing to attend 'The Gift Box' groups rather than do leisure activities. These groups have been run by clinicians I have barely met, who are enthusiastically presenting the outcomes to their colleagues. People who have histories of forensic risk behaviours are feeling safe enough to tell their stories and being more respectful to one another. Other opportunities are opening up, who knows which way it is going to go? My dream is that 'The Gift Box' will continue to develop into a type of 'Recovery College' tool that provides a growth orientation for anyone who co-uses it, enabling relationships that will lead to better mental health and well-being for all (Toney et al., 2018).

I would never have taken any of these steps without the serendipitous meetings, interactions, and support of all the helpful people I met along the track. I would never have even started on this round of my journey of recovery except for Josephine's unfailing encouragement. Each new encounter kept me believing that my renewed sense of pathway was leading somewhere that would be of use to a slightly bigger part of the world than my own small sphere. So far, I haven't reached a dead end, even though, if I had been the author of my own destiny, this would never have been the story I would have written for myself.

EPILOGUE

It's About Time

Meaning and Mattering

Co-creating this duo-ethnography has been enriching and empowering for both Josephine and me. But it has not been easy. Finding ways to write evocatively about our lived and felt experience was sometimes painful. But the overall process has been intellectually challenging and personally engaging.

Josephine's habit, in writing, is to seek feedback. She invited friends and family to read the draft manuscript as it developed. Subsequently, conferring with each other about their feedback was occasionally tricky. One instance occurred when, in an early draft, I had described reading every page of the Bible and coming to love it. Josephine was concerned that my written account of my spiritual journey did not do it justice, but she was struggling to find anything specific to address. One reader told Josephine that the description came across as a wholesale embracing of every word of the Bible. This seemed incongruous to her, considering the range of biblical accounts of the best and the worst of humankind. Josephine's knowledge of the Bible is patchy, but she pulled together some inaccurate stories from her memory, writing comments that questioned what I had made of accounts of child sacrifice, incest, and violence.

I was working on the manuscript in a difficult context at home, with workmen outside. Reading these ill-thought-out comments about an experience that was so precious to me, on this day at this time, sent me into a tailspin. These comments did not feel like an inquiry; they felt like a threat to my reality. I literally felt like throwing my computer out of the window. It was as if the only place I had to stand had been knocked out from under me. There was an echo of being hurled into the abyss with no lifeline – re-covering that old ground of the threat of obliteration.

This was a low point in our joint endeavour. It was an object lesson in the risks we were taking in the duo-ethnographic process of disrupting each other's thinking in the service of developing written text, while writing about such deeply personal experiences. It was not until finalising our conclusions that we were able to talk properly about what happened.

216

Despite my initial reaction at the time, I reflected on my writing in the light of the upsetting comments. It became clear that what I had written had not captured the depth and complexity of my lived experience of reading the Bible – and what it meant to me. Our relationship and the computer survived the challenge. I eventually wrote a much fuller description of the impact that beginning to read the Bible had had. Once Josephine read this version, she had more understanding of the original description. We have often found increased depth of meaning in the same words once we have looked more deeply at the context. It is not unusual for published words to be received in quite different ways from how they were meant. We wanted to ensure as much clarity as possible in conveying our meaning-making to readers.

Ultimately, the feedback proved extremely helpful but the intensity of self-protective rage that I felt let us know we needed to take more care. We still used written feedback but always spoke about it first. Maintaining the connection in the moment by spoken conversation helped progress the meaning-making.

Another example of needing to write more evocatively happened when we were working on my accounts of synchronicity. Josephine had found the stories engaging when I had spoken about them, but in written form they fell flat, like a series of anecdotes without enough interest to hold the reader's attention. She wondered if they could be written more succinctly. In keeping to the publisher's word limit, we had to make every word count.

The story of the ring, on which were engraved the words, *This too will pass,* was a case in point. Initially, in my attempt to describe the impact on me of repeatedly hearing the phrase 'this too will pass' around that particular time, I had written that I was 'astounded by this synchronicity'. Josephine questioned the use of the word *astounded,* as for her, the phrase was a common one.

This felt invalidating. For me, it had been a novel phrase. Meaningful coincidence, or synchronicity, was one of the most important aspects of my life. My initial response was to remove both that and other anecdotes, rather than have my experiences of synchronicity further misunderstood. At least the word count was reduced. However, the issue did not feel resolved. It took some careful and painful conversations, with the support of mutual friends, for us to find a way to move beyond either shortening the anecdotes or taking them out.

The outcome surprised both of us. Rather than writing the accounts of my experiences of synchronicity more succinctly, I rewrote them with more detail. I made my reality stand out, and clarified the importance of the timing and juxtaposition of events that gave them their quality of meaningfulness. This took substantially more words. Both of us felt the longer accounts were more evocative and enriched the book.

Experiencing a sense of meaning in our lives is central to both of us. As for everyone, what we value and find meaningful is intensely individual. It involves living our own unique lives, according to what matters most, in the best way possible. It also involves mattering to others, and having loved ones, companions, acquaintances, and even strangers who matter to us. Contributing to other people's lives also feels important to us. It is our hope that this book will be helpful to all who read it.

One significant threat in finding meaning in life emanates from the interplay of power dynamics. Such dynamics can be seen on a large scale in colonisation, where one culture is imposed on another – in work, education, friendships, marriages, families, and every part of life. In any of these contexts, there is a risk that one party feels pressure to discount their sense of meaning for the sake of a relationship. This is also a risk in the clinical relationship.

People in general usually are not aware of the power they hold. Whether clinicians are aware of it – or choose it, or not – power and rank are invested in the clinical role. The purpose of the clinical relationship is to serve the other person. For clinicians with a focus on service, the idea of holding power is an anathema. However, we need to acknowledge this power and manage it actively in order to be useful to the other person. An important task for us as clinicians is to support the other person to find meaning in their own way.

Over the course of writing this book, Josephine and I have distilled several elements that help us negotiate power dynamics in a way that supports meaning-making. We call these elements 'embracing vulnerability', taking a 'both/and, and beyond' perspective, and 'being with'. Each of these elements has had a place in enabling us to develop our own ways of being ourselves – professionally and personally, and in writing the book. In our view, these factors are also essential for clinical relationships to be healing. Indeed, we believe they have something to offer everyone. I have been interested to find, as we wrote the book, that the tools in 'The Gift Box' incorporate these elements, as they assist in a collaborative meaning-making process.

Embracing Vulnerability

Each of us has vulnerability and we are all wounded in our own ways. There is increasing open discussion of vulnerability, as in the work of Brene Brown (Brown, 2010), and the public acknowledgement of mental health issues by royals, elite sports people, and celebrities. Self-compassion is seen as increasingly important (Neff, 2003). There was little space in Josephine's and my medical training for acknowledging our vulnerability. This is changing; self-care is being taught in medical schools and advocated for doctors and other health professionals (Stillwell, Vermeesch, & Scott, 2017). A New Zealander, Dr Sam Hazeldine, led a petition in 2016 that resulted in a new clause in the Hippocratic Oath, asserting the need for doctors to give priority to our own health as much as to the health of the people we serve.

In 2016, the Australian and New Zealand College of Psychiatry went further than this in publishing an official position statement valuing the contribution of psychiatrists with experience-based expertise. If this had happened

30 years ago, I might have had a different career path, and the doctor patients in our research might have been able to speak openly about the wisdom they acquired from their own mental health journeys.

We welcome this change because we believe that if clinicians (ourselves included) deny our own suffering and vulnerability, we risk a detached clinical treatment process where we engender the belief that 'sick' people are different from us. Embracing our own vulnerability supports us to be available to the people we serve with the same compassion we are showing to ourselves. In some important way, we are all the same.

This phrase, *We are all the same,* came to me in the midst of my first extreme-state episode, prompting me to hug everyone in sight, and to burst into Anthony Ryle's consulting room when he was with someone else. During that extreme state, I had a vision of publishing a book called *It's About Time.* I saw myself as a change agent, travelling on the edge of time in the vanguard of a movement to bring to everybody this awareness of all people basically being the same, and of equal value. This experience created a sense of pathway in my life, bringing meaning and purpose to my extreme-state vulnerability. While writing this book, it felt pivotal for me to include the words, *It's About Time,* in the title. It was only latterly that the title was changed, for practical reasons of discoverability. It was a relief to me to be given the opportunity to include these meaningful words in the hourglass motif on the book cover.

The Re-covery Model, conceptualising life as a spiral, provides a map any of us can use in understanding ourselves. It embraces vulnerability and challenges as universal experiences, which can become opportunities for re-covering old ground in new ways, building resilience as we find meaning and purpose in what has happened to us. This has emerged from my process of working through and integrating lived experience of extreme states, and collaborating with people I have served as they, too, have worked through similar experiences. This is an ongoing project. I am seeking feedback about the experience of implementing 'The Gift Box' resources so that everyone can help improve and develop them. One of our hopes for this book is that people will experience an increasing sense of possibility that they too can speak out and contribute to others through finding meaning and resolution in their own suffering. This can happen for any of us, given the right support. It is a hope described by the doctors in our study.

Taking a Both/and Perspective, and Going Beyond This

The dominance of a meaning-making system is supported by either/or thinking. *You are either with me or you are against me.* Institutionalised meaning-making systems, such as diagnostic systems and psychological theories, can become dominant in structuring the content of clinical conversations. Alternatives are coming forward. *Drop the Disorder* is challenging the role of diagnostic categories (Watson, 2019). The *Power, Threat, Meaning* framework is advocating a different meaning-making system for training clinicians, while supporting people in making sense of what has happened to them (Johnstone et al., 2018).

As well as alternatives, it is important to have a both/and perspective to avoid the sort of dominance which can lead to devaluing one meaning-making system in favour of another. Taking a 'both/and, and beyond' perspective supports a collaborative process of discovery. Neither Josephine nor I want to discard all of psychiatry, medication, diagnostic systems, and biological approaches. We have seen people hurt by being dominated by these approaches. We have also known people to find them helpful. We see the issue as using these approaches in an effectively nuanced way and holding openness to move beyond current practice.

Recovery Colleges are an example of 'and beyond' in providing a different model for moving towards well-being, sharing the knowledge that people with lived experience of extreme states feel they need (Whitley, Shepherd, & Slade, 2019). Open dialogue and other family-based initiatives are supporting families to be part of the solution (Falloon et al., 1982; Seikkula, Alakare, & Aaltonen, 2011). Early intervention services for psychosis are using both medication and psychological approaches. They have altered the use of the diagnostic system, eschewing the term 'schizophrenia'. They are going beyond these approaches, looking for ways to identify those at risk of psychosis, and intervening before its onset (Yung et al., 1998). Enquiry is proceeding regarding the personalisation of antipsychotic treatment (Wunderink, 2019), and recipients' experience of being on and attempting to withdraw from psychotropic medications (Oedegaard et al., 2020). This subject is close to my heart, given my lived experience of the impact of antipsychotic and antidepressant medication.

As clinicians, we may feel as if we are holding a 'both/and, and beyond' perspective, but this may not be the experience of the people we are working with. This is particularly true in the context of institutions and societal cultures that prioritise certain ways of thinking. If we do not act consciously to bring forward the perspective of the other person, our perspective is at risk of dominating theirs. The 'Bridge of Trust' diagram provides a simple illustration of the reality of differences, as well as similarities, in any two parties setting out to build trust, or in group settings. Holding both/and views in mind creates a platform for going beyond.

It is the clinicians' responsibility to find out how our communications are received. We need to ask and find a way for people to tell us. For example, we might ask: 'How is this conversation working for you?' or 'What are you noticing going on in your thinking while I am talking?' The feelometer, now part of 'The Gift Box', provides a practical tool for facilitating feedback.

The hundreds of cards in 'The Gift Box' that identify experiences people have had and could have, also help with negotiating some of these challenges in the clinical relationship. They support embracing vulnerability in demonstrating that other people have experienced extreme states and actions too. In a practical way, this exemplifies how we all have experiences in common, diminishing stigma and shame, and safely validating even the most extreme acts. Thus, it becomes acceptable and possible to begin to articulate the unspeakable and find new ways of managing previously unbearable states.

Choosing cards is a less demanding cognitive process than spontaneously generating descriptions. This is helpful for people caught in emotional distress and vicious cycles, which make it hard to articulate experience. Presenting the broad range of experiences and possibilities for helpful intervention depicted in the cards is a practical demonstration of the existence of many both/and alternatives. The wild cards remind people to identify their own experiences and add the option of going 'beyond' the prompts. There are always more possibilities that none of us has thought of yet. This contrasts with a clinical interview structured to elicit symptoms of diagnoses, or impairments in development, which are interpreted as part of a deficit-based formulation.

We need openness to be aware that we don't know what we don't know, and a breakthrough 'aha' moment may be beyond any of our current meaning-making systems. Humility and learning to sit with uncertainty are needed, if we are not to dominate other people's meaning-making systems.

Being with

I crystallised the idea of 'being with' as crucial to my clinical work. The 'Bridge of Trust' diagram also represents building trust as a mutual, active process of being with one another, embracing similarities and differences, attitudes and values, vulnerabilities, and strengths. Often 'being with' involves a non-verbal, felt connection.

'Being with' in an effective way as a clinician appears deceptively simple but is complex. We need to be attuned to ourselves and the other in order to notice the responses we have, and use them in the encounter in a way that works for the other person. Being with another person in this way, without trying to change our responses or theirs, creates a context which enables meaning-making and makes change possible. To do this effectively requires us as clinicians to own, validate, and normalise the personal, lived experience of each and every one of us.

And yet, training in a clinical role can make it harder to 'be with' the people we serve in a healing way. As clinicians, we have spent many years learning pathologising perspectives. They become part of what equips us to be experts in our practice. As doctors, we are trained to elicit information which will enable us to come to a formulation, diagnosis, and treatment plan. This excludes much of the kind of ordinary conversation any two people use to connect. These concerns are readily identified with respect to doctors, and what is described disparagingly as the 'medical model'. But they are not limited to doctors. Institutional practices, requiring assessment, diagnoses, and treatment plans privilege particular meaning-making systems, which can be stigmatising and disempowering. The power dynamic privileges the knowledge and values of the clinician over those of the person they are there to serve. The expert position does not easily support a healing sort of 'being with'.

Over the course of writing this book, Josephine and I have consistently spent time 'being with' one another. Often, this has taken place on the phone, as we live in different towns. Our attitude towards one another is of openness and curiosity, acceptance, and warmth. Often, we have been quietly present – waiting, listening, and trying to understand while the other spoke. We have done a lot of checking in. We have a powerful commitment to valuing what each other has to say. We have curiosity as to how the other sees things and real interest in hearing about it. At times we have offered words for each other's experiences; some of these have been embraced and some rejected. As we have got in touch with intense emotion or experienced the temporary loss of a meaning that has accompanied transformation, we have known we are not alone.

Our Dream

These challenges apply in everyday interactions for everyone. All of our lives could be immeasurably improved if we could become aware of, and address, the power dynamics in human relationships. 'Embracing vulnerability', knowing on some level that we are all the same and that we all have equal value; taking a 'both/and, and beyond' perspective; and 'being with' one another in healing ways, have the potential to support all of us to function optimally, and to find the meaning and purpose of our lives. Our dream is that everyone will wake to find ourselves in a world where there is no *other*, and we are all *us*.

It's about time.

REFERENCES

Arieti, S. (1964). *Interpretation of Schizophrenia* (2nd ed.). New York: Basic Books.

Bentall, R. P. (2003). *Madness Explained-Psychosis and Human Nature*. London: Penguin Books.

Bochner, A. P., & Ellis, C. (2016). *Evocative Ethnography. Writing Lives and Telling Stories.* New York: Routledge.

Breault, R. A. (2016). Emerging issues in duoethnography. *International Journal of Qualitative Studies in Education*, *29*(6), 777–794. doi:10.1080/09518398.2016.1162866

Brown, B. (2010). *The Gifts of Imperfection: Let Go of Who You Think You're Supposed to Be and Embrace Who You Are.* New York: Barnes and Noble.

Chang, H. (2008). *Autoethnography as Method. [References]: Autoethnography as Method* (229 pp.). Walnut Creek, CA: Left Coast Press.

Crowther, A., Taylor, A., Toney, R., Meddings, S., Whale, T., Jennings, H., … Slade, M. (2019). The impact of recovery colleges on mental health staff, services and society. *Epidemiology and Psychiatric Sciences*, *28*(5), 481–488. doi:10.1017/s204579601800063x

Davidson, L. (2016). The recovery movement: Implications for mental health care and enabling people to participate fully in life. *Health Affairs*, *35*(6), 1091–1097. doi:10.1377/hlthaff.2016.0153

Day, J. C., Wood, G., Dewey, M., & Bentall, R. P. (1995). A self-rating scale for measuring neuroleptic side-effects. *British Journal of Psychiatry*, *166*(5), 650–653.

Deegan, P. (1990). Spirit breaking: When helping professions hurt. *Humanist Psychologist*, *18*, 303–313.

Deegan, P. (1996). Recovery as a journey of the heart. *Psychiatric Rehabilitation Journal*, *19*(3), 91–97. doi:10.1037/h0101301

Ellis, C. (1997). Evocative autoethnography: Writing emotionally about our lives. In W. G. Tierney & Y. S. Lincoln (Eds.), *Representation and the Text: Reframing the Narrative Voice* (pp. 115–139). Albany, NY: State of New York Press.

Ellis, C., Adams, T. E., & Bochner, A. P. (2011). Autoethnography: An overview. *Historical Social Research-Historische Sozialforschung*, *36*(4), 273–290.

Falloon, I. R. H., Boyd, J. L., McGill, C. W., Razani, J., Moss, H. B., & Gilderman, A. M. (1982). Family management in the prevention of exacerbations of schizophrenia – A controlled-study. *New England Journal of Medicine*, *306*(24), 1437–1440. doi:10.1056/nejm198206173062401

Fowler, H. W., & Fowler, F. G. (1982). *The Concise Oxford Dictionary of Current English* (7th ed.). Oxford: Oxford University Press.

Fromm-Reichmann, F. (1950). *Principles of Intensive Psychotherapy*. Chicago, IL: University of Chicago Press.

Geekie, J., Randal, P., Lampshire, D., & Read, J. (Eds.) (2011). *Experiencing Psychosis: Personal and Professional Perspectives*. New York: Routledge.

Greenberger, D., & Padesky, C. A. (1995). *Mind Over Mood: A Cognitive Therapy Treatment Manual for Clients*. New York: Guilford Press.

Groff, S., & Groff, C. (1989). *Spiritual Emergency: When Personal Transformation Becomes a Crisis*. New York: TarcherPerigee.

Illich, I. (1975). *Medical Nemesis: The Expropriation of Health (Open Forum/Ideas in Progress Series)*. Richmond London: Calder & Boyars.

Jamison, K. R. (1996). *An Unquiet Mind*. New York: Vintage Books.

Jaspers, K. (1964). *General Psychopathology* (J. Hoenig & M. Hamilton, Trans.). Chicago, IL: University of Chicago Press.

Johnstone, L., Boyle, M., Cromby, J., Dillon, J., Harper, D. J., Longden, E., … Pilgrim, D. (2018). *The Power Threat Meaning Framework: Towards the Identification of Patterns in Emotional Distress, Unusual Experiences and Troubled or Troubling Behaviour, as an Alternative to Functional Psychiatric Diagnosis*. London: British Psychological Society.

Kapur, S. (2003). Psychosis as a state of aberrant salience: A framework linking biology, phenomenology, and pharmacology in schizophrenia. *American Journal of Psychiatry*, *160*(1), 13–23. doi:10.1176/appi.ajp.160.1.13

Karns, C. M., Moore, W. E., III, & Mayr, U. (2017). The cultivation of pure altruism via gratitude: A functional MRI study of change with gratitude practice. *Frontiers in Human Neuroscience, 11*. doi:10.3389/fnhum.2017.00599

Laing, R. D. (1967). *The Divided Self. An Existential Study of Sanity and Madness*. London: Penguin Books.

Leibrich, J. (Ed.) (1999). *A Gift of Stories. Discovering How to Deal with Mental Illness*. Dunedin: University of Otago Press/Mental Health Commission.

Linehan, M. (1993). *Cognitive Behavioral Treatment of Borderline Personality Disorder*. New York: Guilford Press.

Lovden, M., Wenger, E., Martensson, J., Lindenberger, U., & Backman, L. (2013). Structural brain plasticity in adult learning and development. *Neuroscience and Biobehavioral Reviews*, *37*(9), 2296–2310. doi:10.1016/j.neubiorev.2013.02.014

Markin, R. D. (2018). "Ghosts" in the womb: A mentalizing approach to understanding and treating prenatal attachment disturbances during pregnancies after loss. *Psychotherapy*, *55*(3), 275–288. doi:10.1037/pst0000186

Markman, H., Stanley, S., & Blumberg, S. L. (1996). *Fighting for Your Marriage: Positive Steps for Preventing Divorce and Preserving a Lasting Love*. San Francisco, CA: Jossey-Bass.

Mason, O., & Brady, F. (2009). The psychomimetic effects of short-term sensory deprivation. *The Journal of Nervous and Mental Disease*, *197*(10), 783–785.

Masson, J. M. (2003). *The Assault on Truth: Freud's Suppression of the Seduction Theory*. New York: Ballantine Books.

Mazereel, V., Detraux, J., Vancampfort, D., van Winkel, R., & De Hert, M. (2020). Impact of psychotropic medication effects on obesity and the metabolic syndrome in people with serious mental illness. *Frontiers in Endocrinology, 11*. doi:10.3389/fendo.2020.573479

REFERENCES

McGlashan, T. H. (1984). The chestnut-lodge follow-up-study. 2. Long-term outcome of schizophrenia and the affective-disorders. *Archives of General Psychiatry, 41*(6), 586–601.

Mosher, L. R., Menn, A., & Matthews, S. M. (1975). Soteria – Evaluation of a home-based treatment for schizophrenia. *American Journal of Orthopsychiatry, 45*(3), 455–467. doi:10.1111/j.1939-0025.1975.tb02556.x

Mosher, L. R., & Menn, A. Z. (1978). Community residential-treatment for schizophrenia – 2-year follow-up. *Hospital and Community Psychiatry, 29*(11), 715–723.

Moskowitz, A., Dorahy, M., & Schafer, I. (Eds.) (2019). *Psychosis, Trauma and Dissociation: Emerging Perspectives on Severe Psychopathology* (2nd ed.). Hoboken, NJ: Wiley-Blackwell.

Neff, K. (2003). Self-compassion: An alternative conceptualization of a healthy attitude toward oneself. *Self and Identity, 2*(2), 85–101. doi:10.1080/15298860390129863

Oedegaard, C. H., Davidson, L., Stige, B., Veseth, M., Blindheim, A., Garvik, L., … Engebretsen, I. M. S. (2020). "It means so much for me to have a choice": A qualitative study providing first-person perspectives on medication-free treatment in mental health care. *BMC Psychiatry, 20*(1). doi:10.1186/s12888-020-02770-2

Polese, D., Fornaro, M., Palermo, M., De Luca, V., & De Bartolomeis, A. (2019). Treatment-resistant to antipsychotics: A resistance to everything? Psychotherapy in treatment-resistant schizophrenia and nonaffective psychosis: A 25-year systematic review and exploratory meta-analysis. *Frontiers in Psychiatry, 10*. doi:10.3389/fpsyt.2019.00210

Putman, N., & Martindale, B. (2021). *Open Dialogue for Psychosis Organising Mental Health Services to Prioritise Dialogue, Relationship and Meaning.* London: Routledge.

Randal, P. (1995). Divining psychiatry. *Australasian Psychiatry, 3*(6), 393–397.

Randal, P. (1999). Loving relationship is at the root of recovery. In J. Leibrich (Ed.), *A Gift of Stories. Discovering How to Deal with Mental Illness* (pp. 137–144). Dunedin: University of Otago Press/Mental Health Commission.

Randal, P. (2012). Subjective experience of spirituality and psychosis. In J. Geekie, P. Randal, D. Lampshire, & J. Read (Eds.), *Experiencing Psychosis: Personal and Professional Perspectives* (pp. 57–65). New York: Routledge.

Randal, P., & Argyle, N. (2005). "Spiritual Emergency" – A Useful Explanatory Model? A Literature Review and Discussion Paper.

Randal, P., Geekie, J., Lambrecht, I., & Taitimu, M. (2008). Dissociation, psychosis, and spirituality: Whose voices are we hearing? In A. Moskowitz, I. Schafer, & M. J. Dorahy (Eds.), *Psychosis, Trauma and Dissociation: Emerging Perspectives on Severe Psychopathology* (pp. 333–345). Chichester: Wiley-Blackwell.

Randal, P., Simpson, A. I. F., & Laidlaw, T. (2003). Can recovery-focused multi-modal psychotherapy facilitate symptom and function improvement in people with treatment-resistant psychotic illness? A comparison study. *Australian and New Zealand Journal of Psychiatry, 37*(6), 720–727. doi:10.1080/j.1440-1614.2003.01261.x

Randal, P., Stewart, M. W., Proverbs, D., Lampshire, D., Symes, J., & Hamer, H. (2009). "The Re-covery Model" – An integrative developmental stress-vulnerability-strengths approach to mental health. *Psychosis-Psychological Social and Integrative Approaches, 1*(2), 122–133. doi:10.1080/17522430902948167

Rapp, C. (1998). *The Strengths Model: Case Management with People Suffering from Severe and Persistent Mental Illness*. New York; Oxford: Oxford University Press.

Rosen, A., Wilson, A., Randal, P., Pethebridge, A., Codyre, D., Barton, D., ... Rose, L. (2009). Psychiatrically impaired medical practitioners: Better care to reduce harm and life impact, with special reference to impaired psychiatrists. *Australasian Psychiatry, 17*(1), 11–18. doi:http://dx.doi.org/10.1080/10398560802579526

Seikkula, J., Alakare, B., & Aaltonen, J. (2011). The comprehensive open-dialogue approach in Western Lapland: II. Long-term stability of acute psychosis outcomes in advanced community care. *Psychosis-Psychological Social and Integrative Approaches, 3*(3), 192–204. doi:10.1080/17522439.2011.595819

Shakespeare, W. (2015). *Hamlet*. London: Penguin.

Stanton, J. (1995). Weight-gain associated with neuroleptic medication – A review. *Schizophrenia Bulletin, 21*(3), 463–472.

Stanton, J. (2003). Talking to families about ADHD. *Journal of the American Academy of Child and Adolescent Psychiatry, 42*(12), 1386–1386. doi:10.1097/01.chi.0000091947.28938.1d

Stanton, J. (2005). Talking to families about ADHD. *Journal of the American Academy of Child and Adolescent Psychiatry, 44*(2), 111–112. doi:10.1097/00004583-200502000-00001

Stanton, J., & Randal, P. (2010). Doctors accessing mental-health services: An exploratory study. *BMJ Open, 1*(1), e000017.

Stanton, J., & Randal, P. (2016). Developing a psychiatrist-patient relationship when both people are doctors: A qualitative study. *BMJ Open, 6*(5). doi:10.1136/bmjopen-2015-010216

Stanton, J., & Simpson, A. (2001). Murder misdiagnosed as SIDS: A perpetrator's perspective. *Archives of Disease in Childhood, 85*(6), 454–459. doi:10.1136/adc.85.6.454

Stanton, J., & Simpson, A. (2002). Filicide: A review. *International Journal of Law and Psychiatry, 25*(1), 1–14. doi:10.1016/s0160-2527(01)00097-8

Stanton, J., & Simpson, A. I. F. (2006). The aftermath: Aspects of recovery described by perpetrators of maternal filicide committed in the context of severe mental illness. *Behavioral Sciences & the Law, 24*(1), 103–112. doi:10.1002/bsl.688

Stanton, J., Simpson, A., & Wouldes, T. (2000). A qualitative study of filicide by mentally ill mothers. *Child Abuse & Neglect, 24*(11), 1451–1460. doi:10.1016/s0145-2134(00)00198-8

Stanton, J., Thomas, D. R., Jarbin, M., & Mackay, P. (2020). Self-determination theory in acute child and adolescent mental health inpatient care. A qualitative exploratory study. *PLoS One, 15*(10), e0239815.

Stillwell, S. B., Vermeesch, A. L., & Scott, J. G. (2017). Interventions to reduce perceived stress among graduate students: A systematic review with implications for evidence-based practice. *Worldviews on Evidence-Based Nursing, 14*(6), 507–513. doi:10.1111/wvn.12250

Sweet, M. (2009). Deregistered psychiatrist is reconvicted for murder of former boss. *BMJ, 338*, b1911. doi:http://dx.doi.org/10.1136/bmj.b1911

Tolle, E. (2005). *A New Earth*. New York: Penguin Putnam.

Toney, R., Elton, D., Munday, E., Hamill, K., Crowther, A., Meddings, S., ... Slade, M. (2018). Mechanisms of action and outcomes for students in recovery colleges. *Psychiatric Services, 69*(12), 1222–1229. doi:10.1176/appi.ps.201800283

Watson, J. (2019). *Drop the Disorder! Challenging the Culture of Psychiatric Diagnosis Paperback*. Monmouth: PCCS Books.

Whitley, R., Shepherd, G., & Slade, M. (2019). Recovery colleges as a mental health innovation. *World Psychiatry*, *18*(2), 141–142. doi:10.1002/wps.20620

Williams, P. (2012). *Re-thinking Madness. Towards a Paradigm Shift in Our Understanding and Treatment of Psychosis*. San Francisco, CA: Sky's Edge.

Wilson, A., Rosen, A., Randal, P., Pethebridge, A., Codyre, D., Barton, D., … Rose, L. (2009). Psychiatrically impaired medical practitioners: An overview with special reference to impaired psychiatrists. *Australasian Psychiatry*, *17*(1), 6–10. doi:http://dx.doi.org/10.1080/10398560802579351

Wunderink, L. (2019). Personalizing antipsychotic treatment: Evidence and thoughts on individualized tailoring of antipsychotic dosage in the treatment of psychotic disorders. *Therapeutic Advances in Psychopharmacology*, *9*. doi:10.1177/2045125319836566

Yung, A. R., Phillips, L. J., McGorry, P. D., McFarlane, C. A., Francey, S., Harrigan, S., … Jackson, H. J. (1998). Prediction of psychosis – A step towards indicated prevention of schizophrenia. *British Journal of Psychiatry*, *172*, 14–20. doi:10.1192/s0007125000297602

INDEX